HOMEOPATHIC REMEDIES

FOR
HEALTH PROFESSIONALS
AND
LAYPEOPLE

HOMEOPATHIC REMEDIES

FOR
HEALTH PROFESSIONALS
AND
LAYPEOPLE

Dale M. Buegel, M.D.
Blair L. Lewis, P.A.-C.
Dennis K. Chernin, M.D., M.P.H.

The Himalayan Institute Press
Honesdale, Pennsylvania

The Himalayan Institute Press
RR 1 Box 405
Honesdale, Pennsylvania 18431

© 1978, 1991, 1999 by The Himalayan International Institute
of Yoga Science and Philosophy of the USA

9 8 7 6 5 4 3 2 1

The cover was designed and illustrated by Jeanette Robertson.
The manuscript was typed by Dale M. Buegel and Blair L.
Lewis. Typesetting and graphics by Blair L. Lewis and
Sandeep Menon.

The paper used in this publications meets the minimum
requirements of American National Standard for
Information Sciences–Permanence of Paper for Printed
Library Materials, ANSI Z39.48-1984.

Library of Congress Catalog Card Numbers: 78–102966

ISBN 0–89389–177–0

Contents

Section 3   *Materia Medica*

Section 4   *Repertory Graphs*

ACKNOWLEDGMENTS

The authors would like to express their gratitude to their families, teachers, and patients. This work would not have been possible without these people.

Our sincere thanks to our teachers of homeopathy, Dr. S. Rama; Rudolph Ballentine, M.D.; Francisco X. Eizayaga, M.D.; Mr. George Vithoulkas, and the teaching faculties of the International Foundation for Homeopathy and the National Center for Homeopathy.

We would like to extend a special thank you to David Kent Warkentin, P.A., and his staff at Kent Associates. His homeopathic computer programs, MacRepertory© and Reference Works©, were valuable in compiling the information used in this book.

Fred Bishop of the International Foundation for Homeopathy; Tori Hudson, N.D., of the National College of Naturopathic Medicine of Portland, Oregon; and John Clarke, M.D., of the Himalayan Institute assisted us greatly in the editing of this book. Copy editing was completed by Betty Buegel, Geneva Boissonnault and David Heitzman.

As always, our families gave us their generous support and love so that this book could be written.

Our thanks to all.

In Service,

Dale M. Buegel, M.D.
Blair L. Lewis, P.A.-C.
Dennis K. Chernin, M.D., M.P.H.

INTRODUCTION

In 1978 when the first printing of this book was released, the resurgence of homeopathy was in its infancy. At that time, we believed it was vital to provide a text for families and individuals that would allow them quick access to treating acute and minor ailments homeopathically. Twenty-one years later, this need is stronger than ever. As homeopathy becomes a mainstream treatment, more people—both laypeople and health professionals—are using homeopathy at home and at work. People are fascinated when they see the results of providing homeopathic care in their own homes. The first time you see Arnica Montana instantly resolve a bad bruise and its associated soreness, homeopathy will find a new friend.

We offer this book to the new and old friends of homeopathy. Learning to integrate homeopathy into your choice of treatment modalities will be an interesting experience. But do remember that, as with any medical treatment system, the scope of problems that homeopathy can address is limited. Each homeopathic prescriber must also acknowledge the limit to the scope of problems he or she can handle. It is important to recognize when the limits of the treatment system or the limits of the prescriber's knowledge have been reached. If the expected result is not forthcoming, seek the advice of those more expert in medical care than yourself.

Thank you for allowing us to participate in your study of homeopathy. We wish you success and good health in this, as in all you do.

Blair L. Lewis, P.A.-C.

Section 1

Principles of Homeopathy

BASIC PRINCIPLES OF HOMEOPATHY

The tradition of homeopathic medicine is long and distinguished. Knowledge and utilization of the "Law of Similars" goes back to the Ayurvedic physicians of ancient India and to the ancient Greek physicians such as Hippocrates. Samuel Hahnemann was a German doctor who rediscovered and systematized homeopathy in the early 1800's. Homeopathy was introduced in America in the 1820's, and by the turn of the century 20-25% of all medical doctors practiced homeopathy. Many medical schools were homeopathic, including four schools in Chicago and the University of Michigan in Ann Arbor. Between 1910 and 1920 homeopathic popularity waned due to complex social, economic, and political reasons. Also, with the advent of antibiotics, heralded as a quick 'cure-all,' a large market for expensive chemical drugs was discovered, and the interest in homeopathy lessened.

While there are only several hundred practicing homeopaths currently in the United States, the number of young physicians interested in homeopathy has grown rapidly. Many other countries practice the art and science of homeopathy. In India and Mexico there are several homeopathic medical schools. Great Britain and West Germany have many homeopathic hospitals and in the East European countries of East Germany, Romania, and Russia, homeopathy is accepted by the state along with the allopathic drug system. In South America homeopathy is also becoming an established practice.

In France, there are thousands of physicians practicing homeopathy and the remedies are sold in almost every pharmacy. Homeopathy is taught at Bordeaux Medical School and University of Pharmacy (Lyon). Because there are no homeopathic medical schools today in the United States, training in homeopathy comes after traditional medical training and residency. Doctors generally learn by apprenticeship with a practicing homeopathic physician. Today, homeopathic medical practices and holistic alternative therapies continue to grow as more and more people are willing to take more responsibility for their own health and wish to use less toxic treatment methods when possible.

One of the basic principles known by ancient physicians and reverified by Hahnemann was that those substances which could produce symptoms in the patient could, with proper preparation, be used to treat those same symptoms. Hahnemann experimented with Cinchona Officinalis (Peruvian Bark), of which one of the active ingredients is commonly known as quinine. He found that if a small amount of his bark preparation were taken every day by healthy individuals, they began to develop fever, chills and a general symptom picture of malaria. He carefully noted the symptoms arising in these research subjects, including such details as the time of the chill, the time of the fever, whether perspiration was associated with the fever or chill, whether the perspiration felt warm or cool, what odor it had, and how the person felt emotionally, as well as detailed observations about every organ system of the body.

Hahnemann, through his training, also knew that quinine was a treatment for malaria, and thus recognized in this treatment approach the Law of Similars, that like could be used to cure like. In other words, that a remedy that produced a certain symptom picture in healthy people could be used effectively for patients whose illness expressed itself in a similar set of symptoms. The symptom picture he obtained was derived according to what was called the Law of Proving, meaning that a healthy subject ingesting a medicinal substance over a period of time will develop a symptom picture related to that particular remedy.

In experimenting with quinine, Hahnemann also developed the Law of Potency. He found that on making an alcohol extract of the bark, diluting this extract 100-fold, and then succussing the preparation (a vigorous method of shaking), the healing properties of the original compound could be enhanced while undesirable side effects were reduced. Hahnemann repeated the process of dilution and succussion again 100-fold, thus having a second potency diluted 10,000-fold from the original extraction. The potencies were numbered according to this dilution schedule, so that the first 100-fold dilution was labeled "1c" (for one centesimal dilution), the second 100-fold dilution was labeled "2c," and so on. He repeated the process as many as 18 times (or an "18c" dilution).

What surprised Hahnemann was that the preparation still had a therapeutic effect. He observed that cures with higher potencies were often more dramatic and more free of the undesirable side effects than when the crude substance was used. He also found, however, that to treat a case, the pattern of symptoms of the patient had to very closely match the symptoms of the proving picture. For example, if the fever and chills occurred at a different time from the time in the proving, the potentized remedy would often not work.

Because of the high dilutions used, many physicians disagreed with Hahnemann's method of treatment. Hahnemann's reputation grew, however, as his treatment results proved far superior to the treatment methods of the time.

To understand how a medicinal substance may have therapeutic benefit with little or no drug present, one must understand the essential nature of the human organism. One way to look at the organism is to identify the different levels of organization and expression present within it. There is the physical level, normally identified as our body, which includes its anatomy, biochemistry and physiology. There is also the level of our mind, dealing with the mental-emotional organization. Between the levels of the physical and mental-emotional organization, many systems of medicine in the world identify a level of organization involving an energy field. Many healing methods have been developed throughout the world, both in ancient as well as in modern times, involving therapeutic effects that appear to act through this energy representation of the organism.

When a person is ill, there may be a disturbance on the physical, mental-emotional, as well as the energy level. The organism responds to this disturbance by trying to heal itself.

The disturbance may result from emotional stress, environmental stress, pollution, bacteria, viruses, nutritional imbalance, or any number of other possibilities. The symptoms that develop, known as the "illness," can be viewed as the organism's best attempt to put itself back in balance. Homeopathy seeks to facilitate the response of the organism to heal itself and restore balance, rather than merely to give drugs to suppress symptoms.

During a cold, for example, mucus production is often the result of the reaction of the body to throw off an undesirable organism and restore physiologic balance. A homeopathic remedy might facilitate this response and foster drainage. An antihistamine would dry up and suppress this response. If one suppresses the drainage through the use of an antihistamine, the human organism may or may not have another way of handling the infection and, at the same time, may have an undesirable reaction to the antihistamine in terms of side effects or toxicity.

Homeopathy should not be viewed as a treatment which will replace all other forms of medical treatment. Homeopathy, like any other treatment tool, has both its advantages as well as its limitations when compared to other treatment methods. Its ability to improve the energy level of the patient, leading to an improved physical-mental-emotional state, is one of the great therapeutic benefits of homeopathy. The physiologic and mental-emotional re-balancing and gradual return to homeostasis may take place over days, weeks and months, even after a single dose of the appropriate remedy.

SELECTION OF THE REMEDY

The first step in selection of a homeopathic remedy for a case is to carefully evaluate the signs and symptoms of the illness in the individual.

The signs and symptoms must be studied and matched with the remedy which produces these same symptoms in a healthy subject (the proving picture). Helpful data in the selection of remedies includes both the subjective observations of the individual's ailment and the prescriber's observations of their behaviors and other physical signs of disease.

In homeopathic prescribing, there are several classes of symptoms used for selecting a remedy. *Mental-emotional symptoms* are extremely important in homeopathic prescribing. For example, a child with fever may desire to be covered or may desire to be uncovered, depending on the individual. This desire would be a mental-emotional symptom that could be used in helping to select the remedy. Another example would be children throwing temper tantrums; one child is not able to be pacified, compared to another child who desires to be held and comforted.

General symptoms are those factors affecting the whole person. For example, the onset of a cold in a particular individual may tend always to come on in wet weather. The occurrence of illness in wet weather would thus be considered a general symptom.

Modalities are also a class of symptoms in homeopathic prescribing. If a sore throat pain is made better by warm drinks, the modality for the sore throat pain would be "better by warm drinks". The whole person is not made better by the warm drinks, only the specific sore throat pain is made better.

Furthermore, *peculiar or unusual symptoms* help in the selection of a remedy. For example, is the fever characterized by absence of thirst? Does the patient sip only small amounts of liquid even though they are very thirsty? Is the burning sore throat relieved by hot drinks instead of cold? Is the pain of an injury relieved by firm pressure, yet aggravated by touch?

Specific symptoms provide the finer detail in describing the case. An example of such symptoms would be pain in the hip, sore throat or nasal drainage. Of the classes of symptoms in a case, mental-emotional, generals and modalities tend to be most important in the selection of a remedy. Peculiar symptoms are unique and often not many remedies have that particular symptom. This allows the prescriber to narrow the choice of remedies to those that fit the total symptom picture. Specific symptoms, though helpful in describing the case, do not generally determine the final selection of a remedy.

In order to select a remedy, the entire case must be taken into consideration, not just one or two general symptoms. For example, in selecting a remedy for a fever, the following symptoms or observations may be helpful: probable cause (exposure to cold, dry winds; exposure to sun; teething); sudden *vs.* gradual onset; restless *vs.* lying still; accompanying delirium or not; accompanying desire to be carried; thirst *vs.* thirstless;

thirst for large or small quantities; perspiration *vs.* no perspiration; relieved by *vs.* unrelieved by perspiration.

Another example would be symptoms or observations important for selecting sore throat remedies: probable cause; gradual *vs.* sudden onset; accompanying confusion, dullness or restlessness; right *vs.* left-sided pain; left-sided pain extending to right; right-sided pain extending to left; sensation of dryness yet moist mouth; aggravation by cold drinks *vs.* warm drinks; relief by warm drinks *vs.* cold; pain improved by swallowing; pain extends to ears on swallowing; accompanying swollen neck glands; painful neck glands; sensation of lump on swallowing; sensation of splinter on swallowing.

Taking all one's symptoms and observations into consideration, one is then ready to find a remedy using the Clinical Repertory and Materia Medica sections of this book.

HOMEOPATHIC REACTIONS AND THE SECOND PRESCRIPTION

The skill of the prescriber can be an important factor in treatment response. In prescribing for oneself or one's family, one should never hesitate to seek more expert advice when necessary.

After the initial prescription, observing and interpreting the reactions to the remedy is a very important and complicated process, especially in chronic cases. For acute cases, however, observation is less confusing, and it is thus easier to decide whether the proper prescription has been made. The classic homeopathic reaction in chronic disease is a slight aggravation of physical symptoms with simultaneous improvement in the internal mental state. Later, improvement of the physical symptoms also occurs.

In transient acute cases, however, the reaction more frequently seen is improvement without an initial aggravation. Sometimes this improvement is instantaneous. Usually, however, improvement occurs gradually. If improvement is noted, the person should be left alone since no further remedy is necessary.

Another type of reaction occurs when the person gets better for awhile but subsequently improvement stops or the condition deteriorates slightly. If the symptoms are still the same and the remedy matches, then repetition of the initial dose is indicated.

Another response occurs when the symptoms change after giving a dose. In this case, a new prescription may be necessary if the symptoms no longer match the original remedy given.

Some illnesses characteristically follow certain patterns. For example, when treating boils, the initial inflammatory (red, hot) stage may require Ferrum Phos. Once swelling commences, Kali Mur may be necessary. Then Silicea may be necessary to bring the boil to a head and promote drainage.

A second example is found in treating upper respiratory illnesses where symptoms often change very quickly, often within a few hours. Initially, the prescriber may find Aconite 30 fits the symptoms, but twelve to twenty-four hours later Arsenicum 30 may be necessary.

Another reaction relevant to home prescribing is when the person fails to improve, or, in fact, worsens. Most often this is due to incorrect remedy selection but may also be due to a more serious constitutional problem. The person's symptoms may at first improve, but soon relapse occurs. Or, the person may seem to improve physically, but emotionally and mentally seems worse. For example, the burning, sore throat may be less intense after prescription, but the ailing individual feels agitated and irritable. Also, a reaction may occur in which the person becomes progressively worse after the initial prescription. In such cases, the symptoms should be taken again to ascertain whether another remedy is indicated or if the physician is needed for further aid.

A common mistake in homeopathy is over-prescribing. The prevailing, faulty attitude is, "If a little doesn't cure it, perhaps a lot will." If the selection matches the symptoms, only a small dose is necessary. Over-prescribing can cause much frustration by confusing the symptoms as the person worsens. One must treat homeopathic remedies with respect since they can be deep and long-lasting in their effect. They are not dietary supplements. While generally safe, frequent repetition of incorrect remedies may cause proving symptoms or perhaps constitutional change.

RECOMMENDED DOSAGE

Homeopathic remedies are dispensed differently from allopathic prescription drugs. Homeopathic remedies are often in the form of globules. Here, the liquid remedy obtained from succussion is dropped onto lactose or sucrose (sugar globules) by the homeopathic pharmacist. Two to five globules (1 - 2 grains) are given at one time.

Coffee products, strong mints and camphor (menthol) tend to antidote many homeopathic remedies and should not be taken while one is being treated homeopathically.

CARE AND ADMINISTRATION OF REMEDIES

Tinctures are used externally, either as lotions (water/alcohol based) or ointments (petroleum based).

The higher potencies are used internally. Globules and tablets are dissolved on or under the tongue in a clean mouth, free of food, toothpaste, mouthwash, tobacco and other strong substances. The remedies should be kept away from strong light or heat. Remedies in potency are activated as soon as they touch moisture. The globules or tablets should not be handled as there may be perspiration on the hands. They should be poured into the cap of the container and then transferred onto the tongue. The patient is not to eat or drink for 15 minutes before and after taking any of the remedies.

To prevent cross-contamination or antidoting, the remedies should be kept in the containers in which they are supplied, and not transferred to other containers.

HOW TO USE THIS BOOK

Homeopathy is a complex science, and many years of study are required to understand its subtleties. Because of its consistency and easy usability, however, the general public can learn to prescribe homeopathically for minor ailments or in first aid situations before a doctor can be consulted. Careful observation and common sense are the means for proper homeopathic home prescribing.

This book serves only as a guideline for people who wish to assume more responsibility for their family's health. Simple problems can often be handled at home. However, this book and the remedies suggested must not be used as a substitute for the physician. Problems which the family feels are too difficult to handle should be discussed with a physician.

When appropriate, other practical non-medicinal hints have been added to the text. Often illness can be treated naturally, without medicines, by taking certain steps to aid the person's natural ability to recover.

The second section of this book is called, "The Clinical Repertory". In this section, categories of illness are listed alphabetically and appropriate homeopathic remedies are listed under each section. A brief description of each of the remedies' symptoms and characteristics are included.

The third section is called "Materia Medica". Remedies are listed alphabetically and described in more detail. It is a partial summary of the various uses which are listed in the Clinical Repertory. It is included so the prescriber has a more complete picture of the remedy, including mental and physical aspects. Most remedies in the Materia Medica have four subdivisions: (1) the "Characteristics" give the most prominent features of the remedy; (2) the "Modalities" show what factors make the symptoms worse or better; (3) the "Clinical Picture" represents areas of the body for which the remedy is useful and provides the prescriber with additional information for analyzing the case; and (4) the "Uses" is a cross-reference to the Clinical Repertory (Section 2). It is a listing of the various categories of illness in the Clinical Repertory where the remedy was mentioned. *It is important that the remedy cover most of the symptoms of the patient. It is not necessary that the patient have all the symptoms of the remedy.* Finding a match in the remedy for at least three of the patient's prominent symptoms is a good indication of likely benefit from the remedy.

If two remedies seem to fit the symptoms of a sore throat, one should look at the Materia Medica to get an overall feeling of the essence of the remedy, in particular the generalities and the modalities. For example, Bryonia and Belladonna may both fit a particular type of sore throat and headache. By looking to the Materia Medica, one will discover that the patients who should receive Bryonia feel better lying down and want to be left alone. Whereas Belladonna patients are characterized by excessive mental agitation, and lying down may aggravate the ailment.

The fourth section is called "Repertory Graphs". Here the computer-assisted repertorization is displayed in visually pleasing graphs for certain ailments and problem areas. The remedies and the rubrics are taken directly from the commentary in Section 2, "The Clinical Repertory". It is easy to view which remedies are more common for an ailment and to quickly view how many remedies share in the same symptom. Symptom grading is also used and explained.

CONCLUSION

This book was written to help with quick, accurate selection of homeopathic remedies for acute ailments. It is both a quick reference as well as a teaching aid for sixty-nine of the most common remedies used to facilitate healing. Symptom guides (see page 14) containing interview questions will teach you how successful prescribers evaluate the case and select needed remedies.

The book is organized in such a manner as to assist both the beginner and the advanced homeopath in acute prescribing. Nothing in this book is meant to replace nor prevent the reader from seeking professional medical care.

All the homeopathic remedies described in this book can be obtained from any reputable homeopathic pharmacy. For home prescribing the authors recommend 30th potency for most homeopathic remedies. It is important to remember that homeopathic remedies can help you only if used properly. With proper understanding and common sense, you can learn to prescribe successfully.

Section 2

Clinical Repertory

INTRODUCTION

The Clinical Repertory is an alphabetical listing of categories of illness and the appropriate homeopathic remedies. A brief description of each of the remedies' symptoms and characteristics is included. You will quickly discover that remedy selection is based on the experiences and sensations of the patient as well as the prescriber's observations. To ease the task of remedy selection, a Symptom Guide has been added for certain categories.

The Symptom Guide will point out key questions and observations to make when interviewing the patient. With these answers, one can easily read the remedies in that category and select the most appropriate remedy. It is also important to point out that both homeopathy and remedy selection are simplified here for the beginner, and a trained homeopath should be consulted when needed.

SYMPTOM GUIDE

This Guide will point out key questions and observations to make about the patient. Learning to think and observe like a homeopath requires one to characterize the entire phenomenon the patient experiences. Special attention is paid to the mental-emotional symptoms and the "Strange, Rare and Peculiar" ("SRP") symptoms.

"That which is out of the common is usually a guide rather than a hindrance ... That which seemingly confuses the case is the very thing that furnishes the clue to its solution." Sir Arthur Conan Doyle.

The General Guide presented here is to be applied appropriately to all the categories in the Clinical Repertory. Specific Symptom Guides have been created for certain disorders. These smaller guides will help you analyze the finer details about an illness. They will also remind you about other ailments that may occur together, such as headache with fever, ear pain with sore throat, etc.

GENERAL SYMPTOM GUIDE

Did the illness begin with a sudden onset of symptoms or a
  gradual onset of symptoms?
What is the mental-emotional state of the patient?
  Restless, dull, anxious?
  Desiring consolation and sympathy?
  Desiring solitude?
  Desiring to be carried or averse to being touched?
What time of day does the patient feel either better or worse?
Position:
  Better or Worse from sitting, standing, lying?
  Lying on which side?
Location of Pain and Symptoms:
  What is the specific location of the pain?
  Does it radiate or extend to other areas of the body; e.g.,
    throat pain extending to the ear?
Sides of the Body:
  Right or left side of the body?
  Does the pain move from right to left, or left to right?
What is the type, duration, and quality of the pain?
  Burning, gripping, stabbing, stinging?
What is the effect of motion?
  Jarring, walking, running, moving specific parts of the
    body?
What is the effect of drinking fluids? Warm and/or cold
    drinks?
What is the effect of eating food? Warm and/or cold foods?
  Overeating versus fasting?
  Thirsty versus thirstless — for sips or gulps?

ABDOMINAL PAIN
(See also Indigestion)

For successful treatment, the quality and character of the pain must be described and the general symptoms obtained. Abdominal pain may be a symptom of a serious medical condition, and if relief is not obtained with a well-chosen remedy, a physician should be consulted.

SYMPTOM GUIDE

Did the illness begin after an emotional upset?
Is the pain better or worse from bending double (curling up in a ball)?
Is the pain better or worse from arching the back?
Better with hard, firm pressure?
What is the effect of bowel movements and urination?
Is there gas? Does passing gas offer relief?
Is the pain better or worse with hot or cold applications?
Better or worse by motion?
What is the effect of food and drinks?

Concomitants:
    With fever?
    With gas, belching, rectal flatus?
    With constipation?
    With diarrhea?
    With vomiting?
    With menstrual period?

Aconite

Fever characteristic of Aconite accompanying abdominal pain that forces one to bend double though this position does not give relief, unlike Colocynthis.

Arsenicum Album

Burning pain in pit of stomach soon after food, relieved by warm liquids. Sensation of weight like a stone in the stomach.

Belladonna

Cases where relief is attained by bending forward. Abdomen tender, distended, aggravated by the least jar. Skin hot, dry. Often associated with high fever; red, flushed face and extreme mental agitation. Symptoms are of rapid onset.

Bryonia

When the patient lies motionless and the pain is made worse by the least movement, jar or touch, and by heat.

Chamomilla

Stomach is distended and gas is passed in small quantities without relief. Often indicated in teething infants. Better by application of local heat. With Chamomilla colic, one often has hot cheeks, red face and perspiration preceding an attack. Can follow a fit of temper. Feels as if in some place the abdomen would burst through.

Cocculus Indicus

The bowels feel as if the intestines were being pinched between sharp stones, with pain so great that fainting and vomiting may follow. Cutting and burning pain as from an incarcerated hernia, worse after rising from sitting. Irritable and hypersensitive to pain. Colic with rectal flatus. Colic from nervousness and from menses.

Colocynthis

Gripping pains forcing the patient to bend double or press something into the abdomen to obtain relief. Patient is restless and may twist and turn to obtain relief. May be caused by undigested food, cold, or occasionally by a violent emotion such as anger. Some relief from hard pressure (unlike Belladonna), and also from passage of gas. Very commonly used.

Cuprum

Coughs and cramps. Symptoms can be intense and violent, spasmodic pains that start and end suddenly. All symptoms are improved by cold drinks. Violent, contracted spasms of the abdomen and upper and lower limbs, with piercing, distressing screams. Colic which is violent and intermittent. Very distressing after-pains from childbirth, particularly in women who have borne many children.

Ferrum Phos

Associated with menstrual periods and characterized by heat, flushing of face and rapid pulse.

Ipecac

Gripping colic, like a hand clutching the intestines. Cutting pains across the abdomen left to right; particularly after acidic or unripe fruit. Worse by motion; better by rest. Associated with nausea and vomiting. Vomiting does not relieve nausea.

Kali Carbonicum

Indigestion with a weak, empty feeling before eating and feeling bloated after eating. Nausea and nervous sensation when hungry. Sour belching. Everything eaten turns into gas. Craves sweets.

Lycopodium
Stomach seems to swell up with gas immediately after a full meal. Pain is better with passing of gas. Right-sided tenderness and pains. Swollen, tender abdomen.

Magnesia Phos
Useful in colic (pain) of the newborn; gas pain in the umbilical region better with drawing up of legs and bending double. Used when there is amelioration by friction, warmth and belching. Also useful for colic in gout and gall bladder attacks that come on shortly after meals. In such cases, a physician should be consulted.

Natrum Phos
Good for colic of children with signs of acidity such as vomiting curdled milk or cream, or passage of green, sour-smelling stools. Colic from inability to pass gas or belch. May come on after eating.

Natrum Sulph
A great deal of belching and/or passing of gas. Colic. Audible rumbling of wind in the bowels. Worse lying on the left side.

Nux Vomica
Caused particularly by overindulgence in food or stimulants (coffee, highly spiced food). Pinching, constrictive type of pains as if the intestines were being rubbed through stones. Abdomen generally hard and drawn in rather than distended, and sensitive to pressure. Worse on motion; better sitting or lying down.

Podophyllum
Gagging, vomiting and/or empty retching. Weak, empty, sinking or sick feeling in abdomen. Thirst for large quantities of cold water. Gurgling through bowels, then profuse, putrid

stools gush out painlessly. Early morning diarrhea (may have urgency that drives one out of bed), during teething, with hot, glowing cheeks. Profuse watery stool with jelly-like mucus.

ABSCESSES AND INFLAMMATION

An abscess is a form of inflammation that is localized to a small area rather than generalized. If generalized symptoms such as fever, headaches, lethargy or multiple sites of infection are present, a physician should be consulted. An abscess (boil) generally starts as an area of redness followed by swelling and pain. As the fluid collects, pus is formed and gathers at the center of the abscess. This may break open and drain until the pus no longer forms and healing takes place. Once the fluid has started to collect, several measures are taken to help bring the boil to a head and facilitate drainage. One method is to apply warm, moist packs to the area of the boil for twenty minutes several times daily. Temperature of the moist pack should be about body temperature so as not to burn the area.

It is important not to irritate the site of the boil by attempting to squeeze the pus out. This will cause the inner borders of the abscess to break and spread the infection inward, becoming systemic or generalized in nature. Except when wet packs are applied, the site of the abscess should be kept dry, free from irritation such as from clothing and left open to the air as much as possible. One should not cover the abscess with non-porous material as this will not allow oxygen to reach the infection and may lead to a more serious infection. If the abscess is draining, one should cover it with a porous material, such as cotton gauze, which will allow the site to breathe and yet soak up the drainage.

Apis Mellifica

Indicated in the early stages of abscess when the skin suddenly appears like a bee sting with shiny swelling becoming pink, then pale in color. Stinging pains. There is an intolerance to heat, improvement with cold applications, worsening of the pain with slightest touch. Generally a bruised soreness. Some itching.

Arnica

Itching, burning, eruption of small pimples or crops of boils. Sensitivity to touch. Skin may be black and blue and have a bruised feeling. Abscesses and boils do not mature but shrivel and crop up again. The Arnica patient feels bruised and sore. Boils occurring after injury.

Belladonna

Rapid development with radiating redness and throbbing pain.

Ferrum Phos

This remedy should be used if there is evidence of a generalized inflammatory process such as fever or multiple sites of inflammation. It should be used early in the development of an inflammation.

Hepar Sulphuris

Unhealthy skin where an abscess may start from the least scratch. Abscess appears with a small, painful pimple that rapidly ulcerates and begins to enlarge. Later, it is a putrid ulcer surrounded by small pimples. There is an extreme sensitivity to touch with pains being sharp and stabbing or sometimes prickly in character. It becomes worse from cold applications; better with warm applications. There is a tendency to bleed.

Kali Mur

This remedy is used during the second stage of infection when there is swelling and pain, but no pus formation. It should be continued even after the pus has formed if there is continued swelling and pain.

Mercurius Sol

Used after Belladonna when pus has formed. Swollen glands. Thin, green pus. Slow formation of pus; pain worse at night. For tonsillar abscess with putrid breath odor and salivation. Constantly moist skin. Do NOT use with Silica.

Pyrogenium

For threatened systemic spread of abscess. If characteristic fever develops, physician should be contacted immediately.

Silicea

Silicea will help the pus form and a painless boil come to a head or help a draining boil heal. At a 6x potency, it should be given every two hours until the boil begins to drain. Then, gradually tapered over a day or two as the congestion and swelling go down. If the swelling is painful, a different remedy will generally be required first. (Do NOT use with Mercurius Sol.)

Sulphur

Acrid, burning pus.

ASTHMA

The wheezing and difficulty in breathing of asthma is generally a manifestation of a more chronic disease which needs the treatment of a physician. Several measures, however, may help the patient during the acute attack. The patient should remove himself from the precipitant of the attack if this is known, such as certain animals, food, fabrics, types of dust, etc. In general, the person should try to relax, avoiding heavy exertion, cold air and certain foods that may lead to mucus formation. These foods include dairy products, sweets, meat, wheat, oats, and, in some cases, barley and rye.

SYMPTOM GUIDE

Is there a sudden onset of asthma, what time?
What time of day does the patient feel either better or worse?
What is the effect of motion?
   Jarring, walking, running?
What is the effect of drinking fluids? Warm and/or cold
   drinks?
Is the patient thirsty or thirstless; for sips or gulps?
Is the onset from exertion (exercise-induced asthma),
   overeating, weather changes, emotions?
Mental-emotional state of the patient?
Better warm room/warm air?
Better cool room/cool open air?
Are the respirations mainly seen with upper chest movements
   or in the abdomen?
Position:
   Better or worse from sitting, standing, lying?
   Lying on which side?
   Do they spring out of bed when the asthma begins?
Respirations:
   Dry or wet, expectoration easy or difficult,
      watery or stringy mucus? Is there coughing?

Concomitants:
   With fever?
   With gas/belching/flatus?

Antimonium Tartaricum

Acute asthmatic attack with abdominal respirations, unable to move chest. Gagging cough with retching or vomiting. White-coated tongue. Associated cough is very loose and rattling but no mucus can be brought up. If effective, relief should be seen within 45 minutes. May repeat remedy every 5-10 minutes.

Argentum Nitricum

Asthma attacks generally follow unpleasant emotions and are accompanied by fear and anxiety. Spasms of muscles make it difficult to breathe. Can't get breath once starts coughing. Can be triggered by laughing. Coughs up pus-filled mucus. Mucus in larynx can trigger cough, as can irritation under sternum. Hoarseness frequently accompanies the asthma.

Arsenicum Album

Time of attacks is generally just after midnight. There is a great deal of anguish and restlessness and fear of lying down because of feelings of suffocation. Associated with a dry, burning cough and with burning and soreness in the chest. There is little expectoration but, if present, is frothy. Arsenicum is often given after Ipecac during the course of an acute attack. Fears death. Worse in wet, damp weather and near seashore. Feels chilly but wants open window.

Calcarea Phos

Tickling cough, yellow phlegm; worse in morning. Breath short, seems difficult. Hoarseness. Tends to clear throat. Fretful, whining disposition. Worse cold damp weather.

Carbo Vegetabilis

Usually comes on in the evening and is associated with long coughing attacks with soreness and burning in the chest. Worse in open air and after eating or talking. The patient is often old and debilitated. Cough may be spasmodic with gagging and vomiting of mucus. Patient desires to be fanned. Asthma usually comes on after a cold.

Ipecac

There is great anxiety with sudden wheezing, shortness of breath and a feeling of suffocation. There is a sensation of a great weight upon the chest. The burning pains of Arsenicum patients are absent. There is often a cough that causes gagging and vomiting. The cough is constant and the patient feels that their chest is full of phlegm, but none is brought up. The extremities are covered with cold perspiration.

Kali Bichromicum

Asthma worse from 3:00 to 4:00 in the morning. Must sit up and bend forward to breathe. Relief comes when patient raises stringy mucus.

Kali Carbonicum

Wheezing worse between 2:00 and 4:00 or at 5:00 in the morning. Usually associated with anxiety and weakness. Chest feels tight and oppressed. Impossible to lie down. Full of phlegm (Arsenicum has dry wheezing). Often rests on knees with head buried in pillow. Tends to stay immobile (unlike Arsenicum).

Lachesis

Short, dry cough, averse to anything tight around the neck or chest. Sensation of suffocation whenever lying down. Feels relief after coughing up watery phlegm. Often indicated in asthma of adults. Attacks often awaken in the morning or occur on going to bed.

Natrum Sulph

Attacks usually come on around 4:00 or 5:00 in the morning with a cough and expectoration (material coughed up) resembling egg white. Later expectoration is greenish and quite copious. There may be vomiting after eating. The patient is always worse in damp, rainy weather. Often indicated in asthma of children. The patient tends to have loose bowel movements on rising in the morning.

Nux Vomica

Attacks of simple spasmodic asthma brought on by gastric disturbances and especially by overeating. There is some relief by belching and the patient must loosen his clothing. Patient is usually irritable and fiery and will feel a constricted feeling at the lower part of the chest.

Pulsatilla

Often has crisis period before 10:00 p.m. on going to bed. Yellow, green, bland mucus; easy to cough up. Wants open air.

BITES
(See Injuries)

BLEEDING

For chronic bleeding tendencies, external or internal, the advice of a physician should be sought. For any local bleeding, direct pressure should be applied. If bleeding is profuse (such as from trauma) the person should be protected from chill and moved, if possible, to a quiet, comfortable place. Medical attention should be sought as soon as possible.

Aconite
When the blood is bright red and there is panic. The patient is thirsty for ice water.

Arnica
Always given first if bleeding follows injury.

Arsenicum Album
Restlessness, shifting of position and marked exhaustion. These symptoms may indicate a large amount of blood loss, and a physician should be consulted.

Belladonna
Blood is bright red, feels hot and clots readily. The head is usually hot and the face red.

Bryonia
Blood is dark, yet fluid, and usually associated with nausea and faintness when attempting to sit up. There also can be headache. The condition is made worse by the least movement.

Carbo Vegetabilis
Bleeding that is associated with symptoms of collapse such as clammy skin and a great desire for air. May have a steady seepage of blood. These are symptoms of hypotensive shock, and a physician should be sought immediately.

Ferrum Phos
Bleeding of nose, especially in children. Bleeding of skin, in general.

Ipecac
Bleeding comes in gushes of bright red blood associated with severe nausea, dark bluish crescents below the eyes, gasping respirations. Especially indicated if these symptoms are

associated with nosebleed or hemorrhage from the uterus. Immediate medical attention should be sought.

Kali Mur
When the blood is black, clotted or tough. Possible vomiting of dark, clotted, thick blood. Nosebleeds of this type tend to occur in the afternoon.

Phosphorus
Profuse bright red blood from nose, rectum, hemorrhoids, mouth or respiratory tract.

BRUISES
(See Injuries)

BURNS
(See Injuries)

CHICKEN POX

Although this illness may present a very constant picture of physical signs, the constitutional or temperamental aspects of the case must be considered.

Antimonium Tartaricum
If resolving eruption has tendency toward blue scarring.

Ferrum Phos
Generalized inflammation with pain, fever and redness.

Kali Mur
Should be taken as soon as eruptions appear to help diminish scarring. May help prevent the infection.

Mercurius Sol
When there is thick, yellow discharges, offensive perspiration; odorous breath; and the patient is overly sensitive to heat and cold temperatures. In general, the patient appears quite sick.

Pulsatilla
Child mild, tearful and not thirsty.

Rhus Toxicodendron
Most frequently indicated remedy. If there is great restlessness of mind and body. Warm bathing relieves itching.

COLLAPSE AND SHOCK

Shock is used in this text in connection with accidents and operations, and collapse in relation more to "medical" cases. The signs and symptoms of the conditions are ashen grey pallor; cold, clammy skin; rapid and weak pulse; restlessness and shallow respiration. Certain immediate measures should be carried out in cases of shock. The patient should be reassured and fear allayed. They should be kept warm with feet elevated. Homeopathic remedies are of value before medical help is available.

Aconite
If fear is very marked, especially fear of death, in shock of sudden onset. This picture may appear after over-exposure to the sun, as in heat stroke. It may first be preceded by an inflammatory picture of sudden onset.

Antimonium Tartaricum
Respiratory distress of newborn, when there is great rattling of mucus but none can be brought up.

Arnica
When there has been injury or bleeding.

Carbo Vegetabilis
When there is great hunger for air, desire to be fanned. Coldness, particularly of the knees. Cold breath.

CONSTIPATION

This is an indication of a more chronic process and, if persistent, one should see a physician. For temporary constipation, squeeze one-half lemon into 8 oz. of hot water with a pinch of salt and 1 teaspoon honey; drink in the morning just after rising.

COUGH AND CROUP
(See Respiratory Infection)

DENTITION (TEETHING)

Babies often have difficulty with restlessness, irritability, fever, diarrhea and upper respiratory problems when their teeth are coming in. Homeopathy can offer relief for children and anxious parents.

Calcarea Phos
Teething pain worse with warm or cold things in mouth. Whining, fretful disposition. Constantly wants to nurse. Pain before diarrhea of either green, loose, slimy stool or hot, watery stool. Also may have headache and respiratory symptoms.

Chamomilla

Most frequently indicated teething remedy. Great sensitivity and irritability. Demands toys yet throws them about immediately; desire to be carried. Often thirsty; diarrhea; dry cough before midnight.

Coffea Cruda

Teething, with fretful tossing about with anguish. Toothaches with excessive pain, which are better holding cold water or ice in the mouth. The toothache returns as the mouth warms up again. Worse from warm drinks and chewing. Violent, throbbing toothache.

DIARRHEA

This is an acute or a chronic condition. If it occurs in children, one should be sure the child drinks enough so that he or she will not become dehydrated. In chronic or severe cases, the physician should be consulted.

Aconite

Diarrhea brought on by exposure to cold, dry wind or result of fright.

Argentum Nitricum

Emotional diarrhea, especially from fear or anticipation. Aggravation from drinking. Shredded, mucus-filled stools, turning green like mashed spinach.

Arsenicum Album

Severe, burning diarrhea resulting from taking tainted food; associated with vomiting, prostration, restlessness, burning pains and anxiety. Stools are scanty, brown, burning to the skin;

pain with defecation. Desire for hot drinks. Exhaustion after passing stool.

SYMPTOM GUIDE

Diarrhea from fear, anger, or anticipation?
Diarrhea from the weather or temperature extremes?
Is there profuse purging?
Are the stools painful or painless?
What color are the stools?
Does it drive the patient out of bed?
What is the effect of eating and drinking? After milk?
What is the effect with motion and rest?

Concomitants:
    With teething?
    With abdominal pain?
    With exhaustion?

Bryonia
Profuse purging, especially with taking cold drinks or when overheated. Stools are brown, thin, and smell like old cheese. Even when there is little disturbance of the bowels during the day, there is often diarrhea as the patient gets out of bed in the morning (Sulphur). Person is irritable, lies motionless, and wants to be alone.

Calcarea Carbonicum
Summer diarrhea, especially after milk. Worse evening (unlike sulphur). Milk may pass undigested. Otherwise, often green, watery, sour stools, with undigested food.

Calcarea Phos

Pain, worse warm or cold things in mouth. Fretful, whiny disposition.

Chamomilla

Diarrhea associated with teething in infants (see dentition). Hot, green watery; looks like chopped eggs and spinach.

China

Rapid general exhaustion from loss of bodily fluids. Painless diarrhea, worse at night and after eating (Podophyllum is usually worse during the day). Often occurs in hot weather, especially after eating fruit. Yellow, brown watery stool, often of undigested food. Rapid general exhaustion from loss of bodily fluids.

Cocculus Indicus

Thin, yellowish, painless stools only in the daytime. Diarrhea from riding in the car, even the shortest distance. Diarrhea with the sensation of sharp stones rubbing together in the abdomen. Intense rectal pain after passing the stool, pain which may lead to fainting.

Colchicum Autumnale

Extremely painful stools with violent urging. Diarrhea in the hot, humid weather of autumn.

Colocynthis

Frequent, jelly-like stools with colicky pains. Temporary relief from passing stool. Made worse by food or drink. Pains made better by drawing legs up to create firm pressure against stomach or by twisting one's torso.

Cuprum

Violent diarrhea with intense abdominal cramps. Weakness from stool, with restlessness and tossing about.

Gelsemium

General state of exhaustion. Copious, yellow flow from relaxed, uncontrolled anus. Anticipation or warm, wet weather may bring on.

Ipecac

Green, frothy or slimy stools. Gripping pain around the navel. Associated with nausea and vomiting.

Mercurius Sol

Stool is green, bloody and slimy. Pain on passing stool and continues after passing; never-get-done feeling. Often associated with chilliness and sick stomach. Worse at night. Flushed, sweaty, but perspiration doesn't relieve.

Natrum Mur

Diarrhea, when present, can be like water, often with mucus. Often alternates with constipation that has frequent urging, with scant, hard and broken evacuations.

Natrum Sulph

Gushing watery stools accompanied with much gas. Early morning diarrhea, worse after breakfast.

Nux Vomica

From dietary, alcohol, or drug indiscretion. Diarrhea alternating with constipation. Worse in the morning and after a large meal.

Phosphorus

Profuse, painless, leaving the person very weak.

Podophyllum

Gurgling through bowels, then profuse putrid stools gush out painlessly. Early morning diarrhea (which may drive the patient out of bed). During teething, with hot, glowing cheeks. Profuse watery stools with jelly-like mucus.

Rhus Toxicodendron

Diarrhea with bloody mucus; tearing pains down legs; extreme restlessness with fever.

Rumex

The end of a cold or after a cold, brings painless, uncontrollable diarrhea with sudden profuse, foul stool. Diarrhea usually occurs from 5:00 a.m. to 10:00 a.m.

Sulphur

Similar to Nux Vomica but unresponsive to Nux with more general characteristics of Sulphur as indicated in Materia Medica. Diarrhea often drives the patient out of bed at 5:00 a.m. to 6:00 a.m.

Veratrum Album

Diarrhea with vomiting, patient is very chilled. Onset of diarrhea may follow drinking cold fluids on hot day or after fright (Gelsemium, Aconite). Green, profuse watery stool, sometimes with flakes resembling spinach. Podophyllum stools, in contrast, are painless, variable color and more forceful.

EAR PROBLEMS

Simple, acute earache is often from congestion due to colds which can respond quickly to the appropriate remedies. The ear should be treated with caution since inflammation behind the eardrum can also involve the throat and eustachian tubes and can spread its infection to other structures in the head. If pain or drainage does not subside within approximately 24 hours, a physician should be contacted. Pain in the ear can often be helped with eardrops of Mullein or Plantago. If these are not available, most drugstores carry glycerine eardrops. Even a drop of unused vegetable oil such as olive oil can help lessen

---

SYMPTOM GUIDE

Is there a sudden onset of ear pain?
What time of day does the patient feel either better or worse?
Better or worse with warm or cool applications?
Worse on swallowing?
Sensitive to air or drafts?
What is the effect of motion?
    Jarring, walking, running?
What is the effect of drinking fluids? Warm and/or cold
    drinks?
Thirsty or thirstless — does the patient prefer sips or gulps?
What is the mental-emotional state of the patient?
Position:
    Better or worse from sitting, standing, lying?
    Lying on which side -- the painful side?

Concomitants:
    Is there a fever?
    Is there discharge from the ear?
    Is hearing impaired?

the pain of a child's ear in the middle of the night. Eardrops are not a substitute for treating the underlying infection, however.

Aconite
Acute onset, often after a chill or draft, with violent pain. May be better with local application of heat. Ear is red, hot, painful.

Belladonna
Face is red, hot and dry; pain is aggravated by the least jarring. Digging, throbbing pain; heat may give relief. Thirst is absent, even with fever present. Often associated with sore throats and swollen glands.

Calcarea Carbonicum
Rupture is common with fatty-looking bland discharge (like chewed paper). May have fluid-filled vesicle or polyps on the eardrum. Swollen glands, slow to resolve, especially on the back of the neck. Noises in the ears.

Chamomilla
Pain is worse by application of local heat. Child may be very cross and fretful, demanding things, then refusing when offered. Child feels better carried. Pains are very severe — making the patient cry out.

Ferrum Phos
Burning, throbbing earache with sharp, stitching pain. Pulsation in ear and head, with beefy redness of eardrum. Drainage from ear may be bloody. Use for earaches after exposure to cold or wet conditions.

Hepar Sulph

Stitching pain; often starts as a sore throat and spreads to the ear. Desire for ear to be warmly wrapped. Tenderness in the bone behind the ear. Peevish patient; nothing pleases him. Worse in the least draft.

Kali Mur

For earaches associated with white tongue and swollen glands and throat. Cracking noises may be heard in the ears on swallowing or blowing the nose. Deafness from swelling. Congested nose.

Mercurius Sol

Pinching, sharp pains in ear, often extending to cheeks and/or jaw. Made worse by lying in bed. See accompanying symptoms in the Materia Medica (Section 3).

Pulsatilla

Brought on by being chilled after being hot, or after getting wet. Pain is worse from application of heat. Patient weepy, wanting attention and company. Consolation will relieve symptoms for a time. Thirstless.

Silicea

Eardrum can have characteristic appearance of redness around the rim. Useful in earache to complete drainage and restore hearing or help ruptured eardrum heal.

Verbascum

Pain with face ache. Squeezing, cramping, paralyzing face ache in malar bones, which are below the eyes and joining the nose. Affects particularly the left side. Feels worse with change of temperature, especially warm to cold. Worse at night and with cough.

EPILEPSY

One should consult a physician in the event of seizure. Immediate care should be provided to the patient to prevent injury. This may consist of protecting a patient's arms, legs and head so that the patient does not injure himself by swinging against hard objects or surfaces. Place the person on their left side or stomach. Care must be taken that the patient does not vomit and aspirate stomach contents during the episode. Consult a physician immediately.

EYE DISORDERS

Eye problems and injuries can be very serious and result in loss of vision. The ophthalmologist, Emergency Department, and local advanced medical care should always be considered first. The following treatment suggestions are for the minor ailments.

Most foreign bodies can be washed out of the eye using large amounts of plain water. If a sensation of a foreign body remains, one should evert the lid. The upper lid may be everted by placing a thin, round object such as a match-stick handle above the eye, below the eyebrow and bone of the forehead, grasping the eyelashes and pulling them upwards as the patient looks downward. If the object can be seen and it is not imbedded, the moist end of a Kleenex can be used to gently brush the object away from the lining of the eye.

If there is pain or bleeding following the removal of the object, consult a physician. Rinsing the eye with Calendula tincture (diluted 1:20 with water) and apply Calendula ointment to the margins of both the upper and lower eyelid may offer immediate relief until advanced care can be sought.

In general, for trauma to the eye, cover the eye with a clean, moist cloth. If there is bleeding, Calendula lotion should be used (diluted 1:20 with water). For a black eye, Arnica may be used internally followed by Ledum if discoloration persists. Symphytum can help for injuries from a blunt object especially if there is no injury to surrounding tissues such as a black eye or if a sensation of a bubble occurs on opening and closing the lid. For injury to the eyeball itself, after surgical operations, and from irritation from foreign bodies in the eye, Aconite (with Arnica) should be used. For direct injury to the eye, it is best to consult a physician. For chemical injury to the eye, the best treatment is rinsing with water—gallons of it! This is especially true if the substance which has irritated the eye was alkaline. Burns to the eye are best treated with rinsing with Hypericum tincture (diluted with water approximately 1:20). This also may be used after the initial rinsing with a chemical burn. In addition, remedies in tablet form can be taken internally for burns, Cantharis is frequently helpful with burns.

For pus in the eye, plain water or dilute boric acid solution (available in most drug stores as an eye rinse) can be used to keep the area clean.

FAINTING

When someone has already fainted, most cases may be treated by loosening the clothing, keeping the patient horizontal and providing them with fresh air. Often fainting can be averted by sitting in a squatting position either on a chair or by lying on the ground with the knees up. If fainting persists or tends to recur frequently, one should consult a physician.

FEVER

It is important to know how high the temperature is and to take the temperature frequently enough to determine whether it is going up or down. The temperature may be taken under the arm, under the tongue or rectally. Keep in mind that normal body temperature is 98.6 F measured beneath the tongue. Temperature measured under the arm will be one degree lower than when measured under the tongue; temperature measured rectally will be one degree higher than when measured under the tongue. Fever is an indication that the body is responding to illness and it is important in the healing process. To further aid the body in cleansing, drink plenty of fluids such as vegetable broth, water or hot water with freshly squeezed lemon juice and a little honey.

If the temperature is very high (103.5 F or above, measured under the tongue), one should begin sponging. This should be done with lukewarm water and should not be overdone. Start sponging only the forehead and face and observing the effect on the temperature. If the temperature drops to 102 or below, the sponging can be stopped. If more extensive sponging is required, the extremities and torso also may be moistened. Do not attempt to drop the temperature back into the normal range by sponging as this will merely suppress the fever and likely chill the patient.

All patients will be thirsty when the fever becomes sufficiently high. Therefore, remedies that are stated as thirstless during fever, are **not** eliminated from patients who have developed a thirst in the later stages of a fever.

Aconite
Anxiety and restlessness; dry skin; violent thirst; relief from sweating. Brought on by exposure to dry, cold winds, or by overheating (such as sunstroke). Frequent chills.

SYMPTOM GUIDE

Fever of sudden onset or gradual onset?
Restless or dull with fever?
Desires to be carried, or averse to slightest touch?
Thirsty or thirstless, mouth moist or dry?
Is the skin white or red, moist or dry, hot or cool?
Is there shivering or gooseflesh?
Desires to be covered or uncovered?
Chills?
Internal heat with external chill or internal chill with external
   heat?
What time of day does the patient feel either better or worse?
Relief with perspiration or not?

Concomitants:
   Note probable cause: overheating, ear problems, teething,
      flu and throat infection.

Apis Mellifica

Fever often preceded by chill around 3:00 p.m. There is frequently thirst with the chill, but thirstlessness during fever. Fever progresses through the evening and into the night. Perspiration may follow which does not particularly relieve symptoms. Fever is often recurrent.

Arsenicum Album

High fever especially worse 12:00 a.m. to 2:00 a.m. Restlessness yet feels weak with slightest exertion to move.

Baptisia

Marked weakness, hard to stay awake, even with conversation. Tired and feeling bruised all over. Mind restless, body lifeless. Restless mind before delirium or with delirium in fever.

Wandering mind that does not want to remain on one subject for any length of time. Sometimes head and limbs seem separate from body. Mistakes own identity for that of two people. Can fall asleep while attempting to speak. Dull, heavy head, hard to hold up head. Tight, drawn sensation, especially toward the back of the head into the neck, with bruised sensation of brain and back of head. Eyes can be very sensitive to light. Soreness of eyeballs, painful to read, and difficult to move. Hot, flushed face, dark red. Constant desire to move, tries to find a softer spot in the bed. Chilly on going into open air, especially chilled on back and limbs.

Belladonna
May have violent delirium; throbbing pulsation in the neck. Skin is hot and burning; eyes red and glistening. May sweat profusely on covered parts without relief. Little or no thirst.

Bryonia
Patient is made worse by movement and prefers to lie still. Faintness on rising; dry mouth and white, coated tongue. Cold, chilly sensations are predominant. Much thirst for large quantities of water at infrequent intervals. Can have intense headache that is always aggravated by the least movement.

China
Rapid general weakness with tendency to perspire from least exertion, movement or during sleep. Desires to fan self. No thirst during chill or long heat that follows. Wants heat source during chill, but does not feel better when provided. Desires to uncover during heat. Following long heat is profuse sweating with intense thirst. Can have periodic fever, such as every two, or less commonly, every three days.

Eupatorium Perfoliatum

Chill begins often 7:00 a.m. to 9:00 a.m. with headache preceding and insatiable thirst. This thirst rarely continues into the fever. Chill generally begins in the small of the back. May be periodic, first one morning, then again the next evening. Accompanying body aches impel to move but movement provides no relief. Perspiration relieves all symptoms except headache.

Ferrum Phos

Dry heat felt in the face, throat and chest. Quickened pulse. Generally useful in all fevers. There may be a chill associated with the fever in the early afternoon.

Gelsemium

Dull, sluggish, apathetic condition. Patient may be dizzy and drowsy. Walking or picking the child up will worsen the dizziness. Fevers brought on by warm, moist, dry weather, and cool evenings. Absence of thirst. Weak, requires support to sit up. Chills along spine.

Kali Mur

Thick, white coating on the tongue; the least draft of cold air will chill the patient thoroughly. Patient may sit near a fire and be adequately covered but still feel cold.

Phosphorus

Increased hunger with fever.

Pulsatilla

Head feels hot but otherwise chilliness predominates; can have intolerably burning heat at night. Thirstless fever with dry lips. Patient usually very weepy and continuously desires comfort. Comfort may even bring down fever.

Pyrogenium

May commence with pains in the limbs. Perspiration has odor of dead animal. Shivering common at times, accompanied by desire to move.

HAYFEVER

This is generally an indication of a chronic condition requiring a constitutional remedy rather than acute treatment. There is a helpful technique called the nasal wash in which one washes the nasal passages with warm salt water. The proper technique must be learned from an experienced teacher in order not to trap water in the sinuses or eustachian tubes causing irritation. In the meantime, several remedies can help.

Allium Cepa

Much sneezing with irritating, copious, watery drainage dripping from nose and burning the skin underneath. Throat is raw from post-nasal drainage. Lachrymation from eyes is usually non-irritating and profuse, though the eyes may burn. Symptoms are better in cold, open air (except cough which may be triggered by inhalation of cold air) and are worse in a warm room.

Arsenicum Album

Sneezing is violently painful, and there may be a tickle in one particular spot inside the nose, not relieved by sneezing. Profuse, watery discharge which burns the lips. The patient is restless and worried. Made worse by changing weather. May have wheezing.

Dulcamara

Eyes swell and water and then the nose runs, followed by the eyes watering again. Constant sneezing with stuffy nose. Worse in the open air and from dampness. Can arise from contact with newly-cut hay. Patient feels chilled when skin is actually hot. Can come from sudden change of temperature (warm to cold).

Euphrasia Officinalis

Profuse tearing, burning the cheeks. Eyes red, puffy; may have ulceration. Film may form and blurred vision relieved by wiping eyes. Not relieved by warm water (Arsenicum Album or Rhus Toxicodendron). May have stinging, shooting pains. Bland, non-irritating nasal drainage in contrast to eyes. Gags when clearing throat in morning because of profuse drainage.

Gelsemium

Eyes feel hot and heavy; tingling sensation in the nose with violent sneezing. Nose streams particularly in the morning, and the discharge burns nose and wings of nostrils. Mouth and throat dry and burning, yet moist; swallowing can cause pain in the ears. Face is red and hot. Patient may ache all over, with limbs feeling heavy.

Kali Mur

Sensation of swelling associated with white coating on tongue.

Nux Vomica

Prolonged distressing spells of sneezing, especially in bed on first waking. Nose is more apt to be stuffed at night. Irritation of nose, eyes and face, with face feeling as if it were close to a hot iron plate. Patient chilly. Discharge non-irritating.

HEADACHES

Headaches are most often a symptom of more chronic constitutional tendencies than of an acute illness. They are a guide for the treatment of chronic conditions. Some headaches have as precipitating factors excesses of living such as drinking, lack of sleep, poor diet, or constipation. These habits must be corrected rather than suppressing the symptom that results from this condition.

While treatment for the chronic condition is being sought, several remedies can help the acute condition. Also, cold packs or warm packs may be helpful.

Aconite
Sudden, violent headaches as if the skull would be forced out of the forehead, or as if the skull were constricted by a tight band.

Symptom Guide

When is the headache better or worse?
What part of the head hurts?
What activities or positions will make the headache pain better or worse?
What brought on the headache -- food, emotion, lack of sleep?
Is it a migraine (congestive) headache?
What is the character and duration of the pain?
  Boring, pressing, pulsating, etc.?
Which of the following can make the headache pain become better or worse:
    Light, motion, pressure, touch, heat, cold, stooping, rising up, emotions, reading, working?

Concomitants:
  With nausea?
  With dizziness?
  With fever?
  With changes in vision?

Apis Mellifica

Stinging pain like bee sting; head bent backward or bored into pillow; pain often occipital. Aggravated by heat. Alleviated by cold wraps.

Argentum Nitricum

Brought on by emotions, especially fear, anticipation, anxiety. Also from intellectual work. Dizzy from heights. Head feels large. Bones feel like they are separating. Boring pain left frontal eminence of forehead. Head feels better wrapped in a tight bandage. Headache triggered by unpleasant emotion. Can extend to the teeth. Though the person may feel generally better in fresh air, the headache may be aggravated by this. Nausea and vomiting of bile or sour fluid with headache. Light sensitive.

Arnica

For headaches after injury. If headache persists, consult physician.

Belladonna

Throbbing with violent shooting pains driving the patient almost wild. Patient is too restless to lie down. Lights, drafts of air, noise, and jarring are all unbearable. Pain is most often in frontal region on the right side. Patient has flushed face or dilated pupils. Better with warm wraps to the head, bending the head backwards, or firm pressure (like Bryonia).

Bryonia

Bursting, splitting, crushing headache. On attempting to sit up, feels sick and faint. Drowsy, dry, peevish; hot, flushed face. Better lying down. Wants to be left alone and feels better staying motionless. Worse with touch, but hard pressure helps and may lie on painful side.

Calcarea Carbonicum

Headache is worse with any change of weather, from motion, in the open air and from stooping. Head and face feel hot during headache or from mental exertion. Feels better lying still. Pain can radiate from the forehead to the nose, from the temples to the jaws or from the muscles of the back of the neck to the base of the skull. Dizziness and nausea often present with headache.

Calcarea Phos

Peevish, fretful, whiny. Headache worse moving, worse stooping or change of position, better open air or lying still.

Colocynthis

Severe, often left-sided pain; after vexation; worse resting on back and from stooping. Better by firm pressure and from walking. Eyes may show burning tears with headache.

Ferrum Phos

Bruising, pressing or stitching pain caused from a cold or from heat of the sun. Pains are worse on stooping and moving. Pressing a cold object against the spot relieves the pain. Headaches are pulsating and worse on the right side. Patient may feel a rush of blood to the head. Often cannot bear to have the hair touched. Can be used to treat headaches following injuries to the head, especially after failure of cure by Arnica. In such cases, advanced medical care should be consulted.

Gelsemium

Begins in nape of neck and extends over head, settling above eyes. Great heaviness of eyelids and limbs. Hammering at base of brain. Not thirsty. Aggravated by mental effort, heat of sun or tobacco smoke. Pain often begins in the early morning hours and reaches peak in mid afternoon. Urination may relieve.

Ignatia

Often follows anger or grief; made worse by strong odors; head feels heavy, worse stooping, but better bending forward. Feels as if nail driven through it in one spot. Better after urination.

Iris Versicolor

Headaches that come on after a letdown following a period of stress, such as a weekend after a week of study or stressful work. Often preceded by visual symptoms and burning gastric distress. Frontal headache or periodic migraine, right more often than left. Cloudy vision before headache. Can have temporary blindness with headache. Mouth feels greasy and scalded. Much ropy saliva and sweet taste. Burning, acid vomiting with headache. Vomiting often starts in early morning, 2:00 a.m. to 3:00 a.m.

Kali Bichromicum

Sinusitis headaches, usually worse below the eyes and slightly better with pressure. Thick, yellow-green, sticky mucus that is stringy, ropy in appearance. Blinding headache with an aversion to light and noise.

Lachesis

Throbbing headache, worse with change of position or sun. Better with the appearance of discharges, such as nasal mucus or the menstrual flow, etc. Wakes from pain.

Lycopodium

Right-sided head pain with no loss of appetite. Gas may accompany the headache.

Magnesia Phos

Shooting and stinging pains, which are intermittent and come on suddenly. Relieved by warmth. Headache is worse in the occiput and can be constant while attending to mental labor. Especially useful in tired, exhausted, neurotic individuals.

Natrum Mur

Headache worse using the mind and from reading. Throbbing headache often starts in mid-morning (10:00 a.m.) like small hammers. Headache often accompanied by dry sensation of the tongue, feeling like it sticks to the roof of the mouth. Worse from light and noise. Accompanied by nausea and vomiting and intermittent pulse. Can have stitching pains about the eyes, worse moving the eyes (like Bryonia). Premenstrual headache that persists after menses.

Nux Vomica

Splitting headache, as if a "nail were driven into skull". Nausea and sour vomiting. Wakes up with headache or comes on after eating. After over-indulgence in food or alcohol.

Pulsatilla

Periodic headache. Pressure, distension or throbbing; from eating ice cream or rich food; over-indulgence. Patient tends to cry. Consolation may relieve.

Ruta

Headache after eye strain; eyes are red, hot, tired, especially after prolonged close work such as sewing or reading small print.

Sepia

Sharp pain in lower part of brain extending upward, which brings on vomiting. Another pattern is that of throbbing over the eye (usually left) accompanied by flashes of heat in head, especially with motion. Worse from light, noise.

HEMORRHOIDS

This is a symptom of chronic disease and is best treated by a physician. For relief of an acute attack, until help for the chronic tendency can be sought, apply Aesculus and/or Hamamelis ointment externally. Aesculus 6X, 10 drops in water three times daily will help acute flair-ups of most cases. If they bleed, also take Collinsonia 6X, ten drops in water three times daily. Aesculus, Hamamelis and Collinsonia are available at pharmacies that stock homeopathic remedies.

Arnica
For hemorrhoids secondary to trauma (such as horseback riding or childbirth). Also used as a concurrent remedy in most cases.

Kali Carbonicum
Painful hemorrhoids with stitching pains and profuse bleeding. Feels better when sitting on a hard seat. Also relieved by cold. Hemorrhoids often protrude from rectum.

Lachesis
Violet colored hemorrhoids, very sensitive to contact, pain relieved by bleeding.

Nux Vomica
Large hemorrhoids with burning, stinging and constricted feeling in the rectum, as well as a bruised pain in the small of the back. Especially indicated in people who have sedentary habits or use stimulants. The itching hemorrhoids keep the sufferer awake at night. Relieved by cold water. Bleeding piles with constant urging to stool and a feeling as if the bowel has not emptied itself.

Phosphorus
Profuse bleeding.

Pulsatilla
Hemorrhoids, with itching and sticking pains; hemorrhoids after childbirth.

HICCOUGH

Generally a self-limited condition, but for very obstinate cases causing long-standing soreness, use Magnesia Phos.

HOARSENESS

Generally a self-limited condition but may accompany colds and/or some chronic diseases. One of the most important treatments for hoarseness is to rest the voice. Please see section on coughs and colds for remedies having hoarseness as a symptom of these conditions.

Aconite
Good in the beginning of laryngitis, particularly in children. Often associated with fever, chills, and dry skin. Also may have croupy cough.

Arnica
Hoarseness from trauma or overuse, as in yelling or singing.

Calcarea Carbonicum
Painless hoarseness, hardly audible voice, worse in the morning and better by hawking.

Carbo Vegetabilis
Painless hoarseness, particularly when brought on by exposure to damp, evening air. Aggravated in moist, cool weather. Generally worse in the evening, although symptoms present in the morning as well.

Ferrum Phos
Painful hoarseness of singers and speakers. Onset often due to drafts, colds, or wet conditions.

Gelsemium
General state of exhaustion. May whisper but can't utter sounds. Paralysis of vocal cords after emotional upset.

Hepar Sulph
Patient very sensitive to slightest draft; often associated with exposure to dry, cold winds. A remedy for children, as well as singers. Especially good for chronic hoarseness in professional singers.

Ipecac
Also recommended for complete loss of voice from cold or congestion if associated with nausea and vomiting.

Manganum
Chronic hoarseness. Larynx dry, rough, constricted. Hoarseness is worse in the morning and better after hawking up lumps of mucus. Hoarseness is peculiarly made better by smoking.

Phosphorus
Cannot talk because of pain in larynx.

Rhus Toxicodendron
Hoarseness from over-straining the voice, or during influenza when bones ache.

Sulphur

Hoarseness with low voice or absence of voice, especially in morning. Sore throat better with warm drinks.

INDIGESTION
(See also Abdominal Pain)

Indigestion may be acute or chronic. For chronic indigestion, consult a physician. The acute variety is generally due to over-eating, eating too quickly and not chewing the food or eating too many different types or too many incompatible foods at the same sitting.

Correction of eating habits will often prevent the indigestion from occurring. Acute indigestion is generally self-limited. Emotional upset and mental stress such as anxiety, fear, anger, resentment, impatience and overwork will contribute significantly to this disorder. The remedies are only temporary. If such symptoms occur, take note of the emotional life as well as dietary habits.

Arsenicum Album

Burning pain in pit of stomach quite soon after eating that is relieved by warm drinks. Sensation of weight like a stone in the stomach.

Bryonia

Discomfort after eating, like a stone in the pit of the stomach. Belching with burning liquid (waterbrash) in back of throat. Heartburn and dull pain in upper right abdomen not relieved by warm liquids (contrast Arsenicum). Doesn't want to move.

Carbo Vegetabilis
Pain and tenderness in pit of stomach one-half hour after eating. Abdomen feels heavy with bloating, offensive gas (which gives relief). The simplest food disagrees. Belching always occurs with this remedy.

Chamomilla
Gas with abdominal cramping coming on after anger. Red cheeks and perspiration. Bitter taste in mouth. Pain in abdomen. Worse by warmth.

Colocynthis
Bitter taste; abdomen distended. Pain in abdomen; better by warmth, bending double, or twisting.

Ignatia
Sour belching; much flatulence (passing gas) with rumbling in bowels; hiccough. "All gone" feeling and sinking in stomach made better by deep inspiration. Longs for indigestible foods. Often comes on after fright or grief.

Ipecac
Nausea unrelieved by vomiting. Hiccough; gas; clean tongue; much saliva. Often comes on after eating indigestible foods.

Kali Carbonicum
Anxiety felt in stomach. Acidic, upset stomach; nausea that is better while lying down. Excessive gas. Nausea of pregnancy without vomiting, and worse only when walking.

Lycopodium
Easily feels full. Sense of distress in stomach immediately after eating. Much belching. Abdomen swollen, better by passing gas. Can't bear pressure of clothing.

Natrum Mur

Heartburn after eating, especially during pregnancy, with acidic risings from the stomach. Aching, cramping nausea. Can have sinking feeling with sensation of hard object in the stomach. Common remedy for heartburn of pregnancy.

Natrum Phos

Abdominal pain, especially in children with signs of acidity. Gas, unable to release. Worse after eating.

Nux Vomica

Heartburn and gas from over-indulgence in coffee, tobacco, alcohol. Distended abdomen, bloated a few hours after eating. Worse in the morning. Waterbrash. Ineffectual urge to vomit.

Phosphorus

Vomiting after anesthesia. Hunger soon after eating. Hunger with fever. Vomits cold water after it gets warm in the stomach.

Pulsatilla

Bloating with a sensation of having eaten too much. Sensation of a stone in the stomach one or two hours after eating, especially after fats, warm food or drink. Regurgitates food and burps taste of food. Odd cravings for indigestible things or some special food or drink. Thirstless, weepy.

INFLAMMATION
(See Abscesses & Inflammation)

INJURIES

There are many varieties of injuries to the body. Some are intentional such as tooth extractions and surgical operations, but most are unintentional such as cuts, scratches, bruises, sprains and strains, burns, bites and stings. Homeopathic remedies can greatly aid the injured person to recover quickly. The first order of business is a thorough assessment of the injury. Any injury may have superficial manifestations but also create deeper damage to tendons, nerves, blood vessels, bones and organs. If you are uncertain of the extent of injuries, it is best to consult a physician.

After rapid assessment, bleeding should be controlled. In general, this may be done by applying direct pressure to the site of the bleeding with a clean, moist cloth. Occasionally, bleeding is so profuse that other measures such as applying pressure to an artery may be required. For further training, a Red Cross First Aid course should be taken.

For control of pain and swelling, a cold, moist application is useful. Avoid placing ice directly against the skin.

In transporting injured patients, be cautious not to aggravate the injury. Consult a *Red Cross First Aid Manual* or take a First Aid course to learn how to transport injured patients.

This section is divided into five common categories of injury:

A. **Wounds (incised wounds, lacerated wounds, scratches and abrasions)**
B. **Bites, Stings and Puncture Wounds**
C. **Bruises**
D. **Burns**
E. **Sprains and Strains**

A. WOUNDS

Incised Wounds

Skin is cut by a sharp instrument that may have divided not only the skin but also more important structures underneath. Such a wound may require a physician's attention to repair it, particularly if it is a wide, gaping cut or involves deeper structures. This is especially true of wounds of the hands and feet. Careful inspection of even superficial wounds of these parts of the body is important to prevent loss of function.

If the cut involves only the skin and no deeper structures are involved, the injured part should be soaked with Calendula lotion after thorough cleansing with water (soapy water if the edges are dirty). Then a dressing of Calendula ointment can be applied to protect the injury site. This process of soaking and dressing should be done daily until new skin has healed over (more often if the dressing becomes contaminated).

Hypericum ointment or lotion may be used alone or with Calendula.

Some homeopaths feel that Hypericum is more useful in wounds that have unusual pain associated with them. For both Calendula and Hypericum lotions, one teaspoon of the mother tincture is mixed in one pint of water.

Lacerated Wounds

This type of wound is jagged and irregular, with mangled, torn skin. Not only is skin broken, but underlying tissue is damaged from the force of the blow. Frequently the wound has been contaminated by dirt and foreign debris. Arnica should be given orally for the immediate injury and the wound cleansed and soaked well and covered with Hypericum or Calendula dressing. If the wound involves an area rich in nerves (e.g., finger tips), then Hypericum should be given in addition to Arnica, particularly if the pain shoots centrally. Arnica ointment, however, should never be used with open skin wounds.

Scratches and Abrasions

These are superficial but frequently very painful and potentially disfiguring injuries. Here the top layer of skin is rubbed off and often dirt and tar ingrained in the raw skin. Cleansing with cold water of Calendula lotion will help, but in cases where foreign material has been ingrained, a physician should be seen for the necessary treatment to prevent a dirt tattoo. After cleansing, the abrasion can be covered with a Calendula ointment or lotion and/or Hypericum if there is pain.

B. BITES, STINGS AND PUNCTURE WOUNDS

Usually these are of minor significance, but occasionally the wounds can become infected (human or animal bite). In addition, a person may be allergically hypersensitive to the toxin (bee or wasp sting); or a poison may be introduced (snake). Wounds which appear as lacerations should be treated as above.

For snake, severe animal bite or rabid dog bite, contact physician or emergency room immediately. Before the doctor is seen, however, Hypericum can help, especially if there is pain. For snake bite, Ledum is indicated.

Ledum is also indicated for simple bee and wasp stings, mosquito bites and other puncture wounds.

Apis Mellifica

Bites that cause stinging pains. Sudden appearance of swelling or puffiness on any body parts, generally pinkish colored at first but may be more pale as swelling progresses. Quite sore to touch. Relief with cold applications, aggravation by warmth.

Arnica

Helps alleviate soreness of affected area after bites. Can be used for bee and wasp stings that feel as though they are bruised.

Calendula

Lotion or ointment — useful externally to help alleviate pain and decrease risk of infection.

Cantharis

Used after puncture by nettle or when pain is burning.

Hypericum

For internal use after horsefly bites, or when pains travel up the limb, or when fingertips are involved.

Ledum

A few doses will help alleviate pain, swelling and help counteract the effects of poison. Particularly useful when extremities are cold; after puncture by sharp instrument or after injections and shots where area is sore. Usually the first remedy given. May take remedy every 15 minutes for the first hour or two.

Phosphorus

When profuse bleeding accompanies injury.

C. BRUISES

Bruises are the result of injuries from a blow by a blunt instrument to soft parts of the body, leading to swelling, discoloration and pain. Over-exertion also can cause a sensation of being bruised.

Arnica

Useful when muscles or soft tissues are black and blue or are sore from overuse. Should be given first in any injury.

Arnica Ointment

Used if muscle or soft tissue is bruised; should not be used if skin is broken.

Calendula Ointment

Useful if bruise is associated with broken skin.

Hypericum

Especially indicated if injuries or blows occur to fingers, toes or spine, particularly to the tailbone (coccyx) with shooting pains from site of injury.

Ledum

For blows to the eye causing pain, swelling or discoloration (black eye). Useful after injuries that Arnica fails to heal; or if parts affected are cold.

Ruta

Helps alleviate pain and tenderness when bruise occurs on bone (chin, elbow, skull) and pain is felt on surface of bone, particularly in places where tendons attach to the bone. Pain worse with every movement.

Symphytum

For blunt trauma to the eye without injury to surrounding tissue. Can have sensation of a bubble beneath the lid when opening and closing the eye.

D. BURNS

Three Degrees of Burns

First Degree: **Redness and pain; sunburn.**
Second Degree: **Has blisters.**
Third Degree: **Severe, deep burns of all layers of skin and below.**

Immediately remove the patient from the cause of the burn. Remove the affected part from heat or wash off chemical irritant with copious amounts of cool or lukewarm water. Do not scrub the affected parts as skin and underlying flesh may tear away. Immediately cool the area with cool water, not ice.

In very serious burns involving large areas of the body, consult a physician immediately. There are two prominent and very immediate dangers in large burns. One danger is fluid loss into the area as the tissues swell. Keep the patient hydrated if they can tolerate drinking. The second is the swelling itself which may cause problems. If the leg swells, for example, the swelling may cut off circulation to the extremity.

In cases of electrical burns, the skin manifestations may be very deceiving. Extensive tissue damage may occur beneath the surface of the skin without showing much skin destruction. Cantharis should be given immediately, and immediate medical attention should be sought.

Aloe Vera gel can be useful externally to relieve pain and promote healing.

Arnica
Should be given at once. May be repeated as often as needed if it relieves the pain.

Cantharis

After the initial dose of Arnica, follow with a dose of Cantharis to relieve pain. Repeat every ten minutes until relief is obtained. Whenever pain returns, Cantharis should be given again.

Hypericum

Hypericum lotion should be applied externally, particularly in first-degree burns.

Kali Mur

For first and second-degree burns with redness and blisters; especially if there is white or grayish exudate over the wound.

E. SPRAINS AND STRAINS

These injuries are the result of stretching either the muscles or the ligaments too vigorously. Take Arnica internally as soon as possible after the injury and apply ice packs externally to the area (use moist rather than dry applications) to keep down the swelling and help control the pain. Several homeopathic remedies are indicated after the initial Arnica, depending on how the symptoms develop.

Apis Mellifica

Hot, swollen, tender joint; better with cold applications. Worse with touch, pressure. Stinging pain.

Bryonia

Joint becomes painful and swollen, distended with fluid. Particularly indicated when joint is painful on the least amount of movement and does not improve with continued motion.

Rhus Toxicodendron

Indicated for hot, swollen, painful joints. Pain generally is of tearing character; feels better with warm application. Initially, movement is painful, but the pain gets better with motion (in contrast to Bryonia). Gentle rubbing makes the pain better. Restlessness, as change in position briefly relieves pain.

Ruta

Pain feels closer to the bone such as the shin or wrist, and can be associated with hard swelling where the tendon is attached to the bone. Pain is aching in character and is made worse by every movement of the injured part. (For example, each time the muscle is stretched, the injured tendon will hurt.) Patient restless, but not to the degree of Rhus Toxicodendron.

Symphytum

Mainly used for musculoskeletal problems where there is injury with disruption of the outer layer of bone (periosteum) causing pricking, sticking pains and slow healing. Such disruption can occur where there is a fracture, or where the tendon attachment is partially or completely detached from the bone.

MEASLES

This is a highly infectious illness of childhood that usually occurs 9 to 14 days after being exposed to another child with measles. It begins with high fever and lassitude and is followed by a harsh, barking cough; inflammation of the eyes and runny nose. The rash begins three days later, seen first on the face. In the early stages, if measles is suspected, Aconite, Belladonna, or Ferrum Phos should be given if their symptoms are present (see Fever). Most frequently indicated remedies are Gelsemium, followed by Pulsatilla.

Aconite
May be indicated very early in the illness if the fever of Aconite is present, namely high, sudden fever; dry, hot; accompanied by thirst for cold drinks and red face (though pale when rising from a lying position). Fever tends to be worse in the evening and before midnight and preceded by chills. Eyes are often red and cough is often croupy in nature (hard, barking, loud). There is frequently much restlessness with itching and burning of the skin.

Apis Mellifica
Recurrent fever preceded by chill with thirst around 3:00 p.m. and aggravation of fever into the evening and nighttime hours. Fever is thirstless and not accompanied by perspiration. When fever breaks and perspiration does come it does not particularly relieve symptoms. Thirstlessness remains during stage of perspiration. Mental state is often fidgety, feeling worse if remains still.
Eruptions generally have stinging, burning character accompanied with swelling under the eruption. Eruption may feel quite sore and be intolerant of contact. The Apis picture in measles in a very sick child may indicate the more serious course of the illness and consultation with a physician should be sought.

Bryonia
Chest involved with tiresome, dry, painful cough. Headache with dry mouth and intense thirst for cold water. Generally the rash appears late and the disease runs a regular course. Person prefers to lie motionless.

Ferrum Phos
Given for the initial stage of fever, especially when clear indications for other remedies are not yet present.

Gelsemium

Fever is prominent symptom (often thirstless). Very high temperature. Sluggishness, apathy, yet frequently needs to change positions. There is a watery nasal discharge which excoriates the nose and upper lip. Harsh, barking, croupy cough; may have hoarseness. Eyelids droopy and heavy. Should be continued after rash appears, particularly if it is red and itchy. Can have headache at the base of the skull extending to area above eyes. Itching severe enough to prevent sleep.

Pulsatilla

Generally indicated later in the illness when fever has subsided or entirely disappeared. Often has runny nose and eyes with yellow, milky discharge. Troublesome cough and wants to sit up to cough. Child cries easily and wants to be comforted.

MENSTRUAL PROBLEMS

This section addresses a limited range of concerns with menstruation which include the physical and emotional symptoms of Pre-Menstrual Syndrome. Special attention is paid to ovarian and uterine pain associated with the menses. The prescriber may want to refer to the Abdominal Pain section, as well as other sections related to women's symptoms.

Belladonna

Bearing-down pains, worse lying down, better by standing (opposite of Sepia). Early menstruation of profuse, bright red blood. If flow is darker, it is offensive in odor. Paroxysmal (come and go suddenly) cutting pains in a horizontal direction. If there is inflammation of an ovary, right side is more often affected.

SYMPTOM GUIDE

What is the timing of the menstrual flow? Is it too early or too late?
Is the flow light (scant) or profuse (copious)?
    Are there clots?
    Is the flow dark or bright red?
Is there pain; and if so, when -- before, during, or after the flow?
    What is the type, quality and duration of the pain?
    Does the pain or discomfort change with position, warm applications, cold applications, pressure, motion, exertion?

Concomitants:
    [It is important to note at what time during the menstrual cycle do these symptoms appear. For example, is there breast tenderness before, during or after the menstrual flow?]
    Is there back pain?
    Is there breast tenderness?
    Is there depression?
    Are there headaches?
    Is there irritability?

Bryonia

Marked pain in right ovary, aggravated by touch, extending down to the thighs. Can have profuse dark flow or suppression of flow.

Calcarea Carbonicum

Too frequent and profuse menstrual flow accompanied by pain in the breasts before menses and head sweat with cold feet. Emotional stress increases the flow.

Calcarea Phos

Menses often too early, too long lasting and profuse in slender women prone to spells of low energy. Often indicated in painful menses of puberty. Labor-like pains before and during flow. Uterine spasms after urination or bowel movements.

Carbo Vegetabilis

Depressed with menses. The flow has a strong odor. Feeling of weight in uterus and right ovary. Dragging sensation in the abdomen and in the low back. Pains increase and decrease.

Colocynthis

Gripping ovarian pain, causing to bend double to seek relief. Also relieved by heat and strong pressure. Can be particularly triggered following violent emotion.

Ignatia

Menses dark, frequent and with large amount of flow. Labor-like pains better by pressure, lying on back and by change of position.

Kali Carbonicum

Breasts sore before menses. Flow is premature or weak, acrid, and itching. Constant sensation of bearing down. Soreness in genitals before, during and after menses.

Lachesis

Scant, dark, lumpy, offensive menstrual flow. Pains in the hips with bearing-down pain in region of the left ovary. Pain relieved with onset of menstrual flow. Can't bear tight clothing around abdomen. Throbbing headaches, dizziness, cramps in chest, aching in stomach before menses. Abdominal spasms during flow. Diarrhea before menses with pain.

Magnesia Phosphorica

Pain with gas, forcing patient to double over to get relief. Better with rubbing, warmth, belching, drawing legs up.

Natrum Mur

Menses often late, scanty. Sore breasts before menses. Premenstrual headache that persists after menses. Fluttering palpitations before menses. Backache that is better lying flat on back or better by pressing firmly against back in sitting position. Sadness before menses with heightened irritability, especially when consoled.

Nux Vomica

Dark menses accompanied by retching, abdominal cramps, and fainting, especially if in warm room. Pain in breasts before menses.

Phytolacca

Premenstrual breast pain that forms hard lumps.

Pulsatilla

Delayed start of flow, especially at onset of puberty. Changeable flow, starting and stopping, ranging from dark clots to colorless water. Breasts sore. Cramping pains, can hardly tolerate them. Emotionally distressed and changeable. Feels smothered in a closed room.

Sepia

Bearing-down pain in the abdomen and low back. Organs feel as if forced out through vulva, though some relief on sitting with legs crossed. Worse if standing or walking. Gripping pain as if suddenly seized by a hand. This pain or burning pain may shoot upward. Menses is usually late and scant.

Sulphur

Weak, heavy feeling with bearing-down pains above pubic bone in lower abdomen. Pains may run from groin to back. Can have headaches accompanying the abdominal spasms. Flashes of heat often accompany uterine symptoms.

MUMPS

A common childhood infection before immunizations were common; one-third of cases have no symptoms. In cases where symptoms are present, the patient can have high fever or headache and swelling of cheeks and glands under the ear. Usually occurs two or three weeks after exposure to a case.

Belladonna

An important homeopathic remedy for mumps associated with its typical fever symptoms; throbbing, burning skin, especially on the face, without relief from sweating; and nervous irritability. Glands are swollen, hot and red, very sensitive to pressure and often worse on the right side; pains may extend to the ear. This remedy is also indicated when the swelling suddenly subsides and is followed by a throbbing headache and delirium.

Ferrum Phos

Indicated in initial fever stage.

Kali Mur

Indicated when there is swelling, particularly when pain on swallowing is present.

Pulsatilla

Used when there is involvement of the testicles and mammary glands. Thick coating on the tongue; mouth is dry and patient is without thirst, even with the fever. The patient tends to be weepy and demands constant attention.

Rhus Toxicodendron

Mood is sad (see also Pulsatilla) and there is extreme restlessness with constant desire to change position. Glands under ears are swollen, worse on left side; cheekbones sensitive to touch; jaws crack when chewing. Pains in other joints relieved by limbering up.

NAUSEA AND VOMITING
(See also Abdominal Pain and Indigestion)

Although nausea and vomiting can be symptoms of chronic, deep-seated illness, more often they are transient, coming on quickly after a particular inciting stimulus. The 24-hour or 48-hour "flu" will commonly occur at one time or another in most families.

Moreover, food poisoning comes after eating spoiled food (usually after catered affairs, picnics and dining out). In general, sips of hot water are comforting, as are warm applications to the abdomen. In addition to the nausea and vomiting, the person sometimes has diarrhea. In such a case, give a remedy that fits the whole picture, rather than being distracted by two apparently different conditions.

Aconite

Accompanied by inflammatory picture of Aconite. There is often the sensation of a cold stone in the abdomen unrelieved by vomiting. Vomiting may be brought on by cold liquids.

Frequently has the anxious restlessness of Aconite's mental picture.

SYMPTOM GUIDE

Does the aroma, thought, or sight of food cause nausea or
  vomiting?
Does eating or drinking make the symptoms better or worse?
  What is the effect of warm or cold drinks?
Are there any peculiar sensations in the stomach or abdomen?
  For example, the sensation of a cold stone in the stomach
  after vomiting.

Concomitants:
  Nausea with pregnancy?
  Vomiting with pregnancy?
  Vomiting or gagging from coughing?

Antimonium Tartaricum
Thirst for cold water. Nausea, retching and vomiting, especially after eating. Gagging or choking with cough (compare with Ipecac).

Arsenicum Album
Useful for the bad effects of spoiled food, drinking ice-cold water or eating ice cream. Characteristic prostration, restlessness and burning pain. Nausea with retching. Extreme irritation of the stomach, frequently associated with diarrhea. Temporary relief from warm drinks.

Bryonia
Usually from overeating. Violent pain in abdomen with severe vomiting. Thirsty but water returns as soon as it reaches the stomach. Nausea and vomiting come on as soon as patient sits up; better lying down, perfectly still with limbs flexed. Bitter eructations, with nauseating taste.

Calcarea Carbonicum
Vomiting, especially right after taking milk. Ravenous appetite and thirst. May crave or be averse to milk, but milk disagrees. Craves eggs. Feels sick if eats fat when ill.

Chamomilla
Agitated and angry. Much vomiting; belches smell like rotten eggs. Violent retching. Bitter vomiting. Makes violent efforts to vomit as if stomach would tear. Nausea after coffee.

China
Helpful as an added remedy for the effects of fluid loss including rapid exhaustion. Vomiting of acidic, slimy matter, water, and food tends to be accompanied by watery accumulation in the mouth and other associated symptoms of China.

Cocculus Indicus
Nausea with vertigo and sick headache from riding in airplanes, boats and cars. Better with warmth. Aversion to food, even the smell of food. Tense feeling below the stomach as if the waist were constricted by a tight band. Worse from tobacco smoke. Better with warmth and lying quietly.

Colchicum Autumnale
Nausea, especially in pregnancy. Hypersensitive to odors. Hunger and weakness from vomiting. Nausea, especially in the first months of pregnancy, when finding food offensive.

Disgust at the thought, sight or smell of food. All attempts to eat cause violent nausea and vomiting. The smell of food can create intense nausea which leads to fainting. Violent retching. Better when curled up in a ball.

Colocynthis
Vomiting and diarrhea frequently accompanying colicky pain; pain relieved by pressure and bending double. Pain predominates the picture and should guide the prescriber.

Cuprum
Coughs and cramps. Nausea. Stomach cramps that come and go, with nausea and vomiting. Improves with drinking cold water. Vomiting with cough.

Ipecac
Persistent nausea and vomiting. Vomiting preceded by much nausea. Nausea not relieved by vomiting; often comes after eating rich foods, pastry, pork and foods that are difficult to digest. Tongue usually clear or only slightly coated. Can be accompanied by diarrhea.

Kali Carbonicum
Anxiety felt in stomach. Acidic, upset stomach. Nausea which is better while lying down. Craves sweets. Excessive gas. Nausea of pregnancy without vomiting, and worse when walking.

Natrum Mur
Aching, cramping nausea in the morning. Vomiting of frothy, watery phlegm with morning sickness. Can have sinking sensation with feeling of hard object in the stomach. Desire for salty foods (though may also have an aversion for salt). Averse to eating bread.

Nux Vomica

Sour taste and nausea in the morning after eating. Nux patient generally has overindulged in food. Ailments from mental overwork. Nausea and vomiting with much retching. Difficult to vomit. Sensation of a stone in the stomach an hour after eating.

Phosphorus

Vomits cold water recently drunk after gets warm in stomach. Nausea after strong smells (flowers, chemicals).

Pulsatilla

Like Nux Vomica, the Pulsatilla patient who vomits also suffers from a generalized indigestion. Vomiting of food taken long before. Mood is weepy.

Sepia

Gone, empty feeling. May crave acids and pickles to relieve taste in mouth. Morning sickness relieved by eating.

Sulphur

Sour vomiting mixed with undigested food. May not tolerate milk. Morning sickness of pregnancy without vomiting, but with faint, sick spells mid to late morning and taste like vomitus in mouth. Especially averse to meat at that time.

Tabacum

Death-like paleness of face and sensation of weakness. Persistent nausea, vomiting and vertigo. Worse from rising up and looking upwards. Seasickness with vomiting, worse from the least bodily motion; better on deck in fresh, cold air. Nausea worse from the smell of tobacco smoke. Increased saliva with the nausea, especially in pregnancy. Sinking feeling in the pit of the stomach. Child wants abdomen uncovered, which relieves nausea and vomiting.

PAIN

Pain should not be feared, but understood. It is the body telling you that something is wrong; thus it serves a protective function.

It is not only a warning guide but also aids the physician in making a more precise diagnosis. It is wise not to suppress or dull pain without first correcting the cause. Even if the actual painful stimulus is removed, the underlying causal factor may return.

Indiscriminate use of pain killers leads to suppression of vitally needed symptoms and can easily become habit-forming or have unpleasant side effects.

The location, type, intensity and character of pain should be analyzed and used as a guide to the correct remedy. Homeopathic prescription will help alleviate pain by getting at the root cause.

Recurrent pain without a physical cause should be a stimulus to re-examine habits, feelings and modes of expression which may be the cause of the pain.

POISON IVY OR POISON OAK

Reactions to these irritants vary from mild itching to severe systemic problems such as difficulty with breathing. It is important to cleanse the skin thoroughly, immediately after contact with these plants. This may minimize the potential future outbreak of the rash. A preparation called **Technu Poison Oak-N-Ivy Cleanser**® has been found to be very helpful to release the toxin from the skin.

The most useful homeopathic remedy is Rhus Toxicodendron, when relief is possible from wet applications (most often warm). If cold applications feel best, consider

Ledum or Rhus Venenata as possible remedies. If relief is felt with warmth, but aggravated by warmth of the bed, consider Sepia.

POISONING

In any case of suspected poisoning, take the person to the nearest emergency room or call the local poison control center. This center will give you the appropriate first aid instructions. In addition, it is important to find the container so that proper identification and treatment can be made.

RESPIRATORY INFECTIONS

Respiratory infections affect the lining of the respiratory tract (nose, throat, windpipe and lungs). Also, it may involve the eyes, ears and occasionally other body areas such as muscles and joints. There are general symptoms such as emotional changes, change in energy level, fevers, chills, etc. Localized signs and symptoms are also found, such as discharges from nose, throat, eyes, ears, etc.

The categories of respiratory infections covered by this book are croup (a severe, barking type of cough), coughs and colds, sinus infections and sore throats. Fever often comes before respiratory infections, and appropriate remedies from the fever section of the book may be indicated early in the course of illness, followed by other remedies once mucus and later symptoms develop. In addition to the treatment suggested in these sections, one should decrease mucus-producing foods such as dairy products, meat, sweets and grains. Instead, one should eat vegetable broths, fresh juices, teas and fresh fruits.

A. CROUP

This is an acute infection of young children 2 to 4 years of age. It is rare in children under 6 months of age. It usually occurs at night, the child waking into paroxysms of breathlessness characterized by crowing inspiration, barking, metallic cough, husky voice and struggle for breath. The attack lasts one-half to three hours and then eases. It is apt to recur for two to three nights. Both child and parent are usually scared and this tends to aggravate the spasm.

The child should be taken into a bathroom where the shower is running to generate warm steam. If this doesn't relieve the symptoms, the child should be wrapped up and taken into the cool night air or taken into the car and driven with the windows open. If there is still no response, prompt attention at the hospital should be sought.

Several remedies have been found to be of special value in this condition. The most applicable one should be given every two hours until improvement.

Aconite

To be used in the beginning of an attack, especially if there is anxiety or restlessness and tossing about. Attacks generally come on after exposure to dry, cold wind. The child then awakens from sleep that night with a sudden attack. The patient may have hot skin and inflammatory picture of Aconite. Cough is dry, loud and barking without expectoration. Aconite, along with Hepar Sulph and Spongia, are the most frequently used remedies.

Drosera

Barking cough. Cannot recover breathing because of high frequency of coughing. Cannot cough deep enough to obtain relief. Worse after midnight (or early evening and then again after midnight). Vomiting or retching if not able to raise mucus.

Hepar Sulph

Loose, croupy-sounding cough. There may be enough looseness that the child will have choking fits. Pains tend to go from throat to ears, and there may be expulsion of pieces of membrane. Worse upon lying down, in the evening and toward morning.

Kali Bichromicum

Metallic cough. Smothering, oppressive spells that awaken the child choking and gasping. The entire chest heaves with the effort to breathe. Worse from 3:00 a.m. to 5:00 a.m. Violent wheezing with the expectoration of tough, stringy mucus.

Spongia

Croup with dryness of air passages. Cough dry, barking; croup worse with inspiration and before midnight. Wakes with feeling of suffocation. Alleviated by eating and drinking, particularly warm drinks.

B. COUGHS AND COLDS

Coughing usually results from irritation of the air passages. An upper respiratory virus, bacteria, smoking or environmental pollution often initiate the process. Cough is generally a beneficial phenomenon, enabling the lining of the respiratory system to remove the offending agent by forceful expulsion.

Coughing should seldom be suppressed by cough medicines, narcotics or sprays since this may cover up important symptoms needed by the doctor for correct homeopathic prescribing. A cough suppressant may tend to worsen the infection since the material causing irritation cannot be removed by the cough.

Acute coughs, especially those associated with "colds" and sore throats, can be helped by homeopathic home prescribing. More chronic coughs should be evaluated by a qualified physician.

SYMPTOM GUIDE

What is the timing of the cough?
　　Morning, afternoon, evening, in bed, after midnight?
　　Is it constant?
Does the cough wake the patient from sleep or prevent sleep
　　altogether?
How does the weather or room air affect the cough? Is it better
　　or worse with open air, damp air, drafts or warm air?
How does exertion (motion) and position affect the cough? Is it
　　better or worse standing, lying, sitting?
Does the patient hold their chest or head when they cough?
What will cause the cough?
　　Drafts, wind, mucus, talking, emotions, crying, teething?
　　　　Is there mucus?
　　　　Can the mucus be brought up (expectorated) easily or
　　　　with great difficulty?
　　When the patient coughs up the mucus does it alleviate the
　　　　cough?
　　What is the color and character of the mucus?
　　　　Green, white, yellow, ropy, watery, burning, thick?
　　　　Does it make the skin raw?

Types of Coughs:
　　Asthmatic (Wheezing)?
　　Barking (Croupy)?
　　Choking and Gagging?
　　Deep?
　　Dry?
　　Loose and Rattling?
　　Suffocative?

Aconite

Usually given at the first sign of respiratory infection, especially if it comes on after exposure to a dry, cold draft. Frequent sneezing, fever, thirst and restlessness at night. Cough is dry, with a hard ringing sound. Generally only useful during the onset of the infection.

Allium Cepa

Raspy, spasmodic cough without coughing up mucus. Tickling sensation in throat triggers cough. There is a desire to grab the larynx as it tends to ache and, when coughing, feels as if it will tear apart if not held by a hand over the voicebox. Cough can be triggered by inhaling cold air. Person generally feels worse, however, in a warm room and better in cold or open air. Hayfever symptoms generally present.

Argentum Nitricum

Spasms of muscles make it difficult to breathe. Can't get breath once starts coughing. Can be triggered by laughing. Coughs up pus-filled mucus. Mucus in larynx can trigger cough, as can irritation under sternum. Hoarseness frequently accompanies cough.

Arsenicum Album

The hallmark of this remedy is burning pains relieved by heat. Discharges from the nose are thin, watery and burn the skin underneath the nose. There is thirst for small amounts of water. Patient is irritable and restless. Cough is worse lying down and patient feels suffocated. Cough can resemble wheezing of asthma and is generally dry and associated with burning of the chest. Often worse after midnight, awakening the patient.

Belladonna

Patient has red, hot face without relief from perspiration. Violent onset after exposure to chilling, particularly of the head. Dryness is a hallmark of the remedy except for perspiration on covered parts of the body. Cough is dry, tickling and comes in violent paroxysms. When the patient coughs, his head feels as if it will burst. Coughing fits will often end in sneezing or a whoop. The child frequently will cry before the coughing fit begins.

Bryonia

The person requiring this remedy is inclined to lie perfectly still, objecting strongly to being moved and, in fact, will even object to people being in the same room with him. Wants to be left alone. Symptoms are worse with least movement. Patient is thirsty for large amounts of cold liquids, although hot drinks may actually help the cough. The infection tends to travel downward into the chest. Coughing is associated with pain and is hard, dry and spasmodic, shaking the whole body, and is associated with soreness in the chest as well as a "bursting" headache. In such a patient, illness is slow to develop. Nasal discharge is watery; lips and mouth are dry; expectoration, if present, is difficult. Patient feels faint on rising. Cough is aggravated from coming into warm room from cold air. Bryonia picture may appear when drainage no longer occurs.

Calcarea Carbonicum

Cough dry at night, becoming loose in the morning. Notices shortness of breath, palpitations and rush of blood to the chest on exertion. May have partial sweat, especially on the upper chest. Sore to touch, especially under the collarbone. Right lung tends to be affected more often than left. Coughs up yellow, green expectoration, sometimes with blood in it.

Calcarea Phos

Peevish, fretful, whiny. Nose drains in cold room, stuffed up in warm room or outdoors. Sneezing with flow of mucus from nose and increased saliva (may have acid taste). Tickling cough; yellow phlegm; worse in morning. Breath short, seems difficult. Hoarseness. Tends to clear throat.

Carbo Vegetabilis

Indicated in bronchitis with profuse yellow, foul-smelling expectoration associated with difficulty in breathing. Much rattling in the chest and a sensation of burning. Cough begins with itching in larynx and is spasmodic in nature with gagging and some occasional vomiting of mucus. Generally associated with chills and thirst. Occasional exhausting sweats. Desires to be fanned. Often of particular help in old people.

Cuprum

Coughs and cramps. Symptoms can be intense and violent. Spasmodic pains that start and end suddenly. Strong metallic taste (like Mercurius Sol and Rhus Tox). Improves with drinking cold water. Vomiting with cough. Cough in spasms, worse inhaling cool air. Whooping cough. Spasm and constriction of chest.

Drosera

Dry spasmodic, barking cough. Cannot recover breathing because of high frequency of coughing; will use their hands to press against their chest and abdomen to relieve the pain from coughing. Cannot cough deep enough to obtain relief. After midnight (or early evening and then again after midnight). Vomiting or retching if not able to raise mucus. Whooping cough.

Dulcamara

Cough usually follows exposure to cold, wet weather or after becoming chilled when overheated (or from sudden temperature changes from warm to cold). Sneezing is severe, and eyes and nose are generally streaming, although nose alternates being stuffy in cold and runny in warmth, with either clear or yellow discharge. Cough generally loose.

Eupatorium Perfoliatum

Extreme soreness along trachea (windpipe). May hold chest with hands on coughing. Chest feels worse lying on left side. Cough and chest better getting on hands and knees. Worse 2:00 a.m. to 4:00 a.m. Cough excited by tickling in chest. Chest soreness during inhalation. Hoarseness in the morning. Perspiration relieves all symptoms except headache. Body aches impel to move, but movement does not relieve.

Ferrum Phos

Indicated in the first stages of an upper respiratory infection with cough where there is fever.

Gelsemium

Patient feels very sluggish and eyelids appear heavy. Infection usually comes on after exposure to warm, humid weather. Patient has chills, particularly along the spine, and feels alternately hot and cold. Often associated with headache and heavy, aching feeling in the eyelids and limbs. Cough is dry and tearing, associated with a sore chest. As with Bryonia, the patient desires to be left alone, though may request to be moved. Patient has much sneezing, with a feeling of dryness in the nose in spite of an excoriating discharge. Can have a bad taste with dry sensation in the mouth and a thick, yellowish-coated tongue.

Hepar Sulph
Choking, croupy, strangulating cough. Worse being uncovered or eating cold food. Wheezing. Loose cough.

Kali Carbonicum
Bronchitis; whole chest is very sensitive. Wheezing. Asthma or cough attacks between 2:00 a.m. and 4:00 a.m. Sharp, stitching chest pains. Can't lie down; often buries face in pillow while resting on knees instead. Full of phlegm in asthma that is difficult to raise (unlike more dry Arsenicum Album wheezing).

Kali Mur
Indicated if there is a white coating on the tongue. Also indicated if the discharge from the nose or back of the throat is white. Swelling is a major indication — whether it be stuffiness and nasal congestion, closing off the ear canal with resultant fluid build-up in the ear, or swollen tonsils and glands.

Lachesis
Short, dry cough; averse to anything tight around the neck or chest. Sensation of suffocation whenever lying down. Feels relief after coughing up watery phlegm. Attacks often awaken the patient in the morning or can occur on going to bed.

Manganum
Catches cold easily. The slightest cold seems to find its way into the chest. Bones can be sensitive to touch. Pains in various parts of the body, especially the voicebox, often refer pain to the ears. Blowing nose is painful. Cough triggered by such things as sustained talking, loud reading, or peculiarly, by scratching the ear canal. Cough is better while lying down. Hoarseness is worse in the morning and better after hawking up lumps of mucus. Hoarseness is peculiarly made better by smoking.

Mercurius Sol

Cough with yellow or green phlegm, made worse from lying on the right side; worse at night; worse in a warm bed. Much sneezing; nostrils raw with yellow-greenish nasal discharge that smells bad. Perspiring during sleep often occurs.

Natrum Mur

Cough triggered by mucus from post-nasal drainage. Causes hoarseness also. Can also cough from tickling in throat or in pit of stomach (latter often results in bursting headache and sometimes spurts of involuntary urination with cough). Eyes smart, burning, with sensation of sand under the lids. Spasms, sometimes unable to open the eyes. Inflammation with eyes stuck together in the morning. Burning tears. Copious discharge from nose of normal-appearing secretions alternating with dryness. Fits of sneezing. Wings of nose sore, sensitive. Diminished sense of smell and taste.

Nux Vomica

Infection starts from exposure to dry coldness or after overindulgence of food, and is associated with much sneezing with the nose alternately blocked or running. Generally stopped up at night and streaming in a warm room and during the daytime. Non-irritating drainage. Sneezes on awakening. Feels extremely chilly and can't get warm. Shudders after drinking fluids or from the least movement. Alternating chills and fever; excessively irritable. Cough is short, dry and fatiguing; accompanied by headache and soreness in abdominal area.

Phosphorus

Cough worse dry weather, changes of weather, cold air, talking or lying on left side. Sensation of a weight on the chest.

Pulsatilla

Thirstless and peevish; constantly wanting attention or to be held. Infection is associated with thick, yellow, bland discharge in throat, nose and eyes. Worse in the morning. Patient has chills up and down the back. Used in later stages of respiratory infection.

Rhus Toxicodendron

Cough worse from midnight to morning, during a chill or when putting hands out of bed. Usually associated with influenza with aching bones and extreme restlessness. Demands frequent change of position.

Rumex

Dry, tiring, continuous cough triggered by irritation under the breastbone (sternum). Burning in voicebox or windpipe. Hoarseness worse in evening. Can hawk up tenacious mucus. Catches cold from least exposure. Worse from all forms of cold. Seeks warmth.

Sepia

Dryness of voicebox and windpipe, tickling in either of which can trigger cough. Dryness sufficient to cause hoarseness. Cough brings up yellow-green, putrid or salty mucus, usually in morning and evening with some relief in afternoon and at night. If cough occurs at night, can be with suffocation and retching, which weakens one. Can be worse lying on left side.

Spongia

Used in coughs associated with dryness of the air passages and burning of the larynx. Larynx is sensitive to touch. Cough is better after eating or drinking, especially warm drinks. Can be associated with asthma where wheezing is worse in cold air. Awakens with sensation of suffocation.

Sticta

Cold can come on after a sudden change in temperature. Tends to catch cold easily. Cough dry, hacking during the night, can be croupy. Worse inspiration. Prevents sleep. Tickling in larynx or windpipe. Cough can be spasmodic, feels like it can't be stopped once it starts. Pressure or fullness at root of nose. Dry, but constant inclination to blow nose. Incessant sneezing. Dryness, especially back roof of mouth (soft palate). Post-nasal drip makes throat raw.

Sulphur

Not generally first remedy. Persistent accumulation of large amounts of mucus. Worse lying down. Cough in this position may precipitate nausea and vomiting. May have deep voice with hoarseness or absence of voice. Nose stuffed in warm room but unobstructed in open air. Worse covered in bed, will try to uncover. Flushes of heat, especially felt on top of head with feet cold to touch (may feel burning). Often helpful to clear up lingering symptoms.

Tabacum

Hiccoughs and coughs occur together leading to a sense of suffocation. Dry cough with hiccoughs during or after the cough. May vomit with the cough. Intense hiccoughs, as if one would suffocate. Cannot take a deep breath.

Veratrum Album

Dryness of the nose, palate, mouth and throat. Tickling deep in trachea or chest excites cough. Cough worse with cold food or drink. Pain in side or inguinal ring (upper groin) with cough. May vomit with cough. Worse evening and morning. May have easy expectoration or dryness.

Verbascum

Deep hollow, hoarse, barking cough. Does not awaken from the cough. Cough is better with deep breathing.

C. SINUS INFECTIONS

Calcarea Carbonicum

Headache from forehead to nose. Nose is dry by day, drains at night. Stopped up in warm air or out-of-doors. Nose drains while in cold air. Wings of nose may be thickened and ulcerated. Thick, yellow pus stopping up the nose, which may have an offensive odor like that of manure, rotten eggs, or gunpowder.

Hepar Sulph

Boring, aching pain at root of nose and forehead above eyes, especially when waking from sleep. Worse motion, stooping, moving eyes. Better warmth. Yellow or green drainage from nose. Pains of facial bones on parts being touched. Drawing, tearing facial pains extend to ears or temples. Neck has swollen, tender lymph glands.

Kali Bichromicum

Thick, ropy, yellow-green nasal mucus, may be bloody, can form crusts in the nose. Pressure and pain at the root of the nose and cheekbones. Frontal and maxillary sinusitis. Snuffles of children. Violent sneezing. Obstruction of the nose.

Lachesis

Intense pain in face (maxillary sinus) that comes on when purulent drainage from sinus has stopped. Relief from pain is obtained when drainage restarts. Tends to affect left sinus more than right.

Silicea
Promotes drainage of pus. Useful in sinus infections to complete drainage.

Sulphur
Eyes have red margins and foreign body sensation (like sand or splinter). Worse near heat. Ear is itchy. Nose is stuffed indoors, open outdoors. May have red scabbiness in side wings of nose. Bleeds easily.

D. SORE THROATS

This is a common ailment in children under twelve years of age, although adults also can have it. At this young age, the child cannot always describe the details of the pain. To be a successful prescriber, learn to be a careful observer. In anyone, a sore throat must be treated with respect for it may herald a more serious systemic illness. If prone to sore throats, consult a homeopathic physician for constitutional treatment. In the meantime, keeping the neck covered with a scarf will help to prevent recurrent infections. Gargling with warm salt water helps to reduce the pain. The following remedies, if given promptly, will speed the recovery.

Aconite
Often given in first stage of sore throat which comes on violently, especially after exposure to dry, cold wind. Burning, dry, very red throat. Fever. Hurts to swallow.

Allium Cepa
Raw throat with characteristic hayfever symptoms of watery, irritating discharge from nasal passages. Watery, non-irritating discharge from eyes, and much sneezing.

SYMPTOM GUIDE

Did the sore throat appear suddenly or gradually?
What is the probable cause of this illness?
    Emotions, lack of sleep, weather changes, overuse of the
        voice, etc.?
What is the location and character of the pain?
    Right or left side of the throat?
    Right side then moved to left side?
    Left side then moved to right side?
    Burning, lump, plug, splinter or stinging sensations?
What is the effect of cold or warm drinks?
Is the pain better or worse from swallowing?
Does the pain radiate to the ear on swallowing?

Concomitants:
    Pain in the lymph glands of the neck?
    Ear pain with sore throat pain?

Apis
Stinging. Pains in throat, which is swollen. Absence of thirst. Worse with warm drinks.

Arsenicum Album
Burning pains in throat relieved by hot drinks. Although the patient is thirsty, he or she sips only small amounts of liquids.

Baptisia
Foul odor to breath. Papillae raised and project through white or yellow coating. Edges are deep red. Dry mouth with constant thirst for cold drinks. Flat, bitter taste in mouth. Cannot swallow because of spasmodic pain, frequently can only succeed in swallowing water. Dark red. Tonsils swollen. Soreness. Severe weakness with fever.

Belladonna

Throat is dry and burns like fire. Tonsils inflamed and bright red. Tongue bright red or looks like a strawberry. Averse to liquids because of pain. Face red, hot, with dilated pupils. Patient's mood is restless, agitated, sometimes delirious.

Bryonia

Dryness, scraped, constricted feeling is worse coming into warm room. Lips dry. Tongue coated white. Desire to be motionless and left alone. Very thirsty for large amounts of water.

Calcarea Carbonicum

Achiness in morning, worse with swallowing and may extend down the esophagus to the stomach on swallowing. Contracted sensation in the throat. Often also has chronic swelling of tonsils. Swollen glands.

Cantharis

Burning in mouth, pharynx and throat. Blisters in mouth and on tongue. Great difficulty swallowing liquids. Throat feels like fire.

Ferrum Phos

Throat sore, dry, red, inflamed, with much pain. Throat burning with pain. Associated with fever.

Gelsemium

The sore throat develops slowly over several days, often with exposure in warm, moist, relaxing weather. Sluggishness is the hallmark of this remedy. Tonsils swollen and throat feels rough and burning. Swallowing causes pain in throat and ear. May have pain in neck muscles extending up to an area just behind the angle of the jaw near the ears. Usually no thirst. Chills up and down the back. Exhausted, may be dizzy if carried or walking.

Hepar Sulph
Sore throat with well-established "cold." When swallowing, there is a sensation of a splinter or fish bone caught in the throat. Pain on swallowing shooting from throat to ear. Very irritable and sensitive to the least draft. Better with warm drinks.

Ignatia
Feeling of lump stuck in throat. Sensation worse between swallowing, though swallowing is painful. Small yellowish-white ulcers on tonsils. Suits particularly the over-dramatic patient.

Kali Mur
When swelling of the glands and tonsils sets in. Throat ulcerated with white or grayish patches. Tongue coated white. Often useful when no other clear picture of a remedy can be found. Often indicated in thrush (yeast) infestations of mouth and throat.

Lachesis
As if lump in throat; worse on left side. Hot drinks aggravate. Cold drinks soothe the pain. Worse swallowing liquids; pain goes to ear on swallowing.

Lycopodium
Right-sided pain that is relieved by hot drinks. Inflammation of throat and palate with dryness. A sensation of constriction and swelling.

Mercurius Sol

Raw, smarting throat. Foul breath. Thirst and sensation of dryness despite moist mouth and much salivation. Thick, yellow coating on tongue. Painful swallowing but must swallow because of increased saliva. Indentation from teeth on sides of tongue.

Nux Vomica

Rough, scraped feeling. Tickling after waking in morning. Often comes on after overeating the night before. Pain shoots into ears.

Phytolacca

Dark bluish-red appearance. Tonsils swollen. Shooting pains into ears upon swallowing. Cannot swallow anything hot.

Sulphur

Hoarseness with low voice or absent voice; pain is better with warm drinks.

SKIN DISEASES

These are generally manifestations of chronic disease and should be treated as such by a physician.

Apis

Sudden appearance of pink or pale swelling; may progress to purplish color if deeper structure is involved. Severe, sudden itching, stinging, burning sensation and soreness. Feels better with cold applications.

Rhus Toxicodendron

Itching with small fluid-filled bubbles (vesicles) grouped together in clumps with surrounding inflammation. Red and swollen eruptions, like chicken pox or poison ivy. Itching better with warm applications. Rhus Venenata (or Vernix) is similar but has the opposite modality of being better with cold applications and worse with warmth.

Urtica Urens

Prickly heat rash with sweatiness and small vesicles. Prickly burning with swelling and severe itching, worse cold applications and bathing or washing. Hives are smaller than Apis. Apis is also better with cold, not worse.

SPRAINS AND STRAINS
(See Injuries)

STINGS
(See Injuries)

STYES

Styes are infections of the glands lining the eyelids, resulting in small pustules embedded in the eyelids. Generally, moist applications are useful in either bringing the stye to a head or in assisting drainage once the stye has come to a head. These should be applied several times a day for twenty minutes or so.

Apis Mellifica

Styes with sudden, piercing, stinging pains are typical of Apis. Eyelids swollen, red. Better cold applications.

Ferrum Phos

For the initial signs of inflammation where there is redness of the eyelid margin but no swelling.

Hepar Sulph

Sensitive styes, better with warm applications.

Kali Mur

When swelling of the lid has begun.

Pulsatilla

Eyelids inflamed; often stick together; discharge creamy and yellowish. Styes especially on upper lid. Most important is the typical temperament and modalities of weeping, peevishness and changeable moods.

Silicea

To help painless swelling form a head. Continue dosage until stye drains.

TEETHING
(See Dentition)

TOOTHACHE

Dental hygiene is of utmost importance in overall health. Diet is an important aspect in the prevention of tooth decay. Refrain from use of refined sugars and grains. Fresh green vegetables (raw and cooked), whole grains, beans, fresh fruit and dairy products are indispensable. Brushing, gentle dental flossing and gum massage with a clean forefinger are also important, as are regular checkups with a dentist.

Arnica
Useful before and after tooth extraction and dental work, or after injury to the teeth.

Arsenicum Album
Teeth feel sore and long; burning pain; worse after midnight; relieved by warmth to affected area.

Belladonna
Throbbing pains in teeth associated with dry, hot face and restlessness.

Calcarea Carbonicum
Sensitive to chewing. Pain worse at night. Subject to slow tooth eruption or to rapid decay.

Chamomilla
Teething children who are cross and complaining. Toothache after warm drinks, relieved by cold drinks and ice.

Coffea Cruda
Violent throbbing toothache. Teething, with fretful tossing about with anguish. Toothaches with excessive pain, which are better holding cold water or ice in the mouth. The toothache returns as the mouth warms up again. Worse from warm drinks and chewing.

Ferrum Phos
Swollen cheeks or signs of systemic infection such as fever.

Hepar Sulph

Tender abscess of gum especially with inflammation and tenderness where tooth meets gum or over erupting tooth, especially wisdom tooth.

Kali Mur

If there is swelling.

Magnesia Phos

Intense, shooting pain that is relieved with pressure of hot liquids. Pain is increased by slightest movement and is worse with cold liquids.

Mercurius Sol

Teeth tender and aching with swollen gums. Worse from cold drinks and foods, from chewing. Worse at night and from warmth of the bed. Metallic taste; foul breath. Swelling around the jaw. Beginning abscess (consult dentist or physician).

Pulsatilla

Toothache relieved by holding cold water in the mouth. Worse from warm drinks. Dry mouth without thirst. Peevish, desires comfort.

Pyrogenium

If abscess is suspected, a dose of Pyrogenium can be helpful to prevent systemic spread. If characteristic fever develops, dentist or physician should be contacted immediately.

Rhododendron

Tearing, jerking pains, better with food and warmth, worse before storms. Pain worse in bed.

TRAVEL SICKNESS

Borax
Dread of downward motion (for example, difficulty when the airplane descends to land).

Bryonia
Nausea and faintness upon rising, vomiting of bile and water immediately after eating, warm drinks are vomited. Worse with the least motion.

Cocculus Indicus
Nausea with vertigo and sick headache from riding in airplanes, boats and cars. Better with warmth. Aversion to food, even the smell of food. Tense feeling below the stomach as if the waist were constricted by a tight band. Worse from tobacco smoke. Better with warmth and lying quietly.

Ignatia
Indicated if there is nausea associated with a feeling of trembling and fright.

Nux Vomica
A horrible, queasy nausea, which may be associated with a headache, usually felt at the back of the head or over one eye. Bloated feeling. Much gagging and retching which can produce vomitus. Patient seeks to be warm.

Rhus Toxicodendron
Especially valuable in air sickness. Patient feels faint on attempting to rise. Complete loss of appetite. Can have severe frontal headache. Scalp sensitive to touch. Patient has unquenchable thirst, with dry mouth and throat.

Tabacum

Travel sickness with vertigo and vomiting. Death-like paleness of face and sensation of weakness. Persistent nausea, vomiting and vertigo. Seasickness with vomiting, worse from the least bodily motion; better on deck in fresh, cold air. Nausea worse from the smell of tobacco smoke. Increased saliva with the nausea, especially in pregnancy. Sinking feeling in the pit of the stomach. Child wants abdomen uncovered, which relieves nausea and vomiting.

URINARY PROBLEMS

Some simple things can be done to promote healing of urinary infections (cystitis and urethritis). These can be done in addition to other treatments. Increasing fluid intake helps flush the urinary tract and decreases the population of yeast or bacteria. Vitamin C and cranberry juice can help control bacterial population by encouraging an acidic medium. Vitamin C should not be taken if one is taking sulfa-type antibiotic medication (Bactrim® or Septra®, for example) as the Vitamin C inhibits the action of the antibiotic, and may crystallize the antibiotic in the kidneys.

Proper hygiene after stools is important in preventing contamination of the urinary tract with bacteria. Flushing the area with a spray bottle after urination can help with yeast, as can a baking soda douche (a dilute solution of less than one teaspoon of baking soda per quart of water is recommended for yeast infestations).

Apis Mellifica

Burning, pressing pain worse at the beginning of urination. Frequent, often constant, painful urge to urinate. Child cries from agonizing pain before urinating. Cold helps. Bloody, cloudy, dark, milky, frothy or offensive urine.

Cantharis

Intolerable urge to urinate with cutting pain extending to urethra. Burns before, during or after urination. Pain in bladder at beginning of urination, extending to kidneys. May urinate drop by drop, each drop having agonizing pain. Burning is relieved by heat. Urine acrid, bloody, cloudy, dark or red. Can have sediment or pus.

Equisetum

Constant desire to urinate as if bladder full. Urination does not relieve the urge. Tender bladder, worse pressure. Involuntary urination, dribbling, especially at night. Pain in right kidney. Testicles may ache. Heaviness and aching in bladder which remains after urination. Prickling, cutting pain in urethra after urination. Burning in urethra during or after urination. Mucus in urine (different from Cantharis).

Symptom Guide

Is there a sense of sudden urgency to urinate?
Does urinating relieve the urgency?
Is the amount of urine copious or very slight (scant)?
Does motion or activity make the urgency better or worse?
What part of the urethra or bladder hurts?
What is the character of the pain?
    Burning, cramping, stinging, stitching?
When does the pain occur? Before, during or after urination?
What activities or positions will make the pain better
    or worse? Lying, standing, sitting, walking?
What brought on the urinary problem? Emotions,
    poor hygiene, sexual relations, vaginal infection?
What is the color, odor and clarity of the urine?
    Offensive, cloudy, pale, sediment, bloody, pus-filled?
Is there low back or kidney pain?

Ferrum Phos

Frequent urging to urinate with pain from lower bladder to tip of urethra. Feels urge to urinate immediately in order to relieve the pain. Tends to be worse during the day and worse standing, better lying down.

Kreosotum

Frequent urging night and day to pass large amounts of pale urine. Often bland discharge from genitalia just before urination. Urine burns genitalia on passing. Incontinence with cough, wets bed. Incontinence is worse lying down.

Lycopodium

Frequent urination at night, infrequent and small amount during day. Urine of dark color, may leave red sediment in diaper or bedsheet. When larger amounts passed, may be pale and clear with or without sediment. Foamy urine. May have blood. Pain in back before urination causing crying out. Pain relieved by urination. Common with kidney stones or gravel.

Mercurius Sol

Sudden urge to urinate. Green, pus-filled discharge (suspicious for gonorrhea), especially at night with much burning and swelling of urethral opening. Burning between urination also. May have involuntary urination in bed. Urine can be copious or can come out drop by drop. May have blood in urine.

Natrum Mur

Frequent urging, day and night, often every hour, with large amounts of urine passed. Cutting pain after urination. Can have discharge of mucus after urination. Smarting of genitalia. Abdomen may contract in spasm after urination.

Natrum Sulph

Burning on urination during and after urinating. Frequent urging with scanty urination. On retaining urine, may have pain in the small of the back. Dark urine can have yellow or brick-dust type sediment.

Nux Vomica

Pain before urination, sometimes aborts urge to urinate. Pain can be at base of bladder with painful urination drop by drop. May have burning pain before, during and after urination. Urge to urinate also creates urge for passing stool. Can have a pattern of frequent passage of pale, watery urine with thick mucus passing during and after urination. Urine can be cloudy with dirty yellow or brick-dust sediment. Can have pain in kidney with inability to lie on affected side.

Pulsatilla

Often for urinary symptoms of pregnancy. Frequent or constant ineffectual desire to urinate, associated with paroxysmal pains. Urine may escape if unable to get to bathroom shortly after urge occurs. Worse from exposure to cold or dampness. Worse lying on back. Pain in bladder if urge is postponed. Burning in neck (outlet above urethra) of bladder during urination. Urine burning; cloudy, dark, ammonia-smelling, bloody, mucus, or purulent (pus).

Sepia

Aching pressure in bladder with frequent desire to urinate. Can have involuntary urination during first part of sleep. Offensive, cloudy urine with uric acid sediment.

Urtica Urens

Acrid urine causing itching. Itching, burning genitalia. Useful for attacks of urinary colic from uric acid stones, especially if accompanied by fever.

VAGINITIS

If one is not certain of the organism involved, consultation with a physician is warranted as venereal disease can present as vaginal discharge. Some common venereal diseases can produce serious medical complications long after the discharge is gone. Douching can be quite helpful in controlling discharge and discomfort, once the cause is known. Baking soda douche (less than one teaspoon per quart of water) for yeast, otherwise vinegar diluted with water. Also helpful is to repopulate with lactobacillus by douching with liquid preparation or diluted lactobacillus-based yogurt.

Borax

Thrush. Thick, corrosive, starch-like discharge. Stinging, swollen sensation in clitoris. Sensation of burning in vagina.

Symptom Guide

Is there a sense of itching or irritation?
What will relieve the itch?
   Scratching, warm or cool bathing, walking?
Is there pain or a sensation of heaviness?
   Better or worse from sitting with legs crossed?
Is there swelling and inflammation? Where?
What is the nature of the discharge?
   Watery, slimy, cream-like, lumpy, thick, offensive?
   Acrid, burning, corrosive, stinging?
What is the color of the discharge?
   Bloody, green, white, yellow?
Is the amount of discharge copious or very slight (scant)?
Does motion or activity affect the discharge?
When does the problem occur? At puberty, pregnancy or
   menopause; after sexual relations?

Calcarea Carbonicum

Leucorrhea, when present, is profuse, burning, itching, and may be milky or yellow and thick. Especially indicated for discharges occurring in infants or before puberty.

Calcarea Phos

Weak, empty, sinking feeling in lower abdomen. Cream-like discharge or discharge like egg-white. Burning in vagina with pain in bladder and uterus. Burning may extend up into chest.

Carbo Vegetabilis

Burning, thin discharge with sore ulcerations. Itching discharge. Burning across sacrum and deep in pelvis with discharge. Pains increase and decrease.

Helonias

Heaviness and soreness of lower pelvis with constant voluminous discharge, usually white, like sour, curdled milk, though may be dark and coagulated if blood is present. Discharge causes itching and may produce redness, swelling or ulceration of vulva. Discharge and heavy, sore sensation aggravated by exertion, especially lifting. Soreness in uterus may extend to small of back. May have burning in kidney as well as frequent urging to urinate with urine scalding inflamed tissues.

Ignatia

Corrosive pus-filled discharge preceded by spasms of the uterus.

Kali Mur

Non-irritating, milky-white mucus.

Kreosotum

Lumpy, gushing, offensive, corrosive, burning, yellow-white discharge sometimes with odor of fresh, green corn. Prickling pains between labia. Pain worse with urination. Intercourse painful, may result in bloody discharge. Dragging down sensation in back with outward pressure in genitalia (like Sepia). Unlike Sepia, however, there is relief from motion.

Mercurius Sol

Profuse discharge always worse at night, greenish or thick white, corrosive, itching, with relief of itching from washing with cold water. Swelling, redness and very sensitive to touch. Weakens the person, especially in discharges before puberty.

Natrum Mur

Vaginal discharge, if present, may be thick and transparent or whitish. Discharge is copious and may itch or irritate. If burning, greenish discharge occurs, this may indicate gonorrhea and a physician should be consulted. Pimples may occur on genitalia.

Pulsatilla

Delayed start of flow, especially at onset of puberty. Changeable flow, starting and stopping, ranging from dark clots to colorless water. Cramping pains, can hardly tolerate them. Feels smothered in a closed room.

Sepia

Bearing down pain in abdomen and small of back. Organs feel as if forced out through vulva, though some relief on sitting with legs crossed. Worse if standing or walking. Gripping pain as if suddenly seized by a hand. This pain or burning pain may shoot upward. Yellow-green, offensive, often excoriating discharge.

Sulphur

Flashes of heat often accompany uterine symptoms, as does an aversion to wash the area. Inflammation of genitals with pimple-like eruption. Corrosive, offensive, yellowish discharge with pain preceding.

WOUNDS
(See Injuries)

Section 3

Materia Medica

ACONITUM NAPELLUS
(Monkshood) (Aconite)

Characteristics

This remedy is given at the first sign of colds or sore throats, especially those coming on suddenly after exposure to cold winds or drafts or sudden chill. Shivering generally precedes a sudden fever. Illness comes on suddenly, with great violence, usually in energetic, robust individuals. Discharges are profuse. At the stage of pus formation, the remedy is usually not Aconitum.

The mental state often shows fear and anxious restlessness, and extreme sensitivity to pain. There may be painful inflammation without pus formation. Sudden changes of weather, especially changing to cold, dry, windy weather, may bring on the illness, though illness may also come on from over-exposure in the summer heat. Pains, when they occur can be unbearable and alternate with a feeling of numbness or pins and needles sensation. They are particularly prone to involve face and head. Useful in situations when fear is present (of the dark, going on airplanes, agoraphobia).

Modalities

Worse:	In the evening and night, particularly before midnight; lying on affected side.
Better:	In open air; warmth; rest.

Clinical Picture

Mind:	Great fear, anxiety, restlessness in a person who before this sudden illness has felt quite self-assured, energetic, robust.
Head:	Heavy, hot, bursting, pulsating sensation; worse on rising.
Eyes:	Feel dry and hot; lids swollen.
Nose:	Sensation of dry mucus membrane with profuse watery discharge.
Face:	Red, hot, flushed; becomes pale on rising.
Throat:	Red; dry and constricted; intense thirst for cold drinks.
Abdomen:	May have severe pain forcing to bend double, yet bending double does not relieve the pain as in Colocynthis. May be a sensation of a cold stone lying in the stomach, this sensation persisting after vomiting.
Lungs:	Shortness of breath, hoarse, dry, croupy cough.
Heart:	Pulse full, hard, tense and bounding.
Skin:	Red, hot, dry, burning.

Uses

1. Abdominal Pain
2. Bleeding
3. Collapse or Shock
4. Diarrhea
5. Ear Problems
6. Eye Disorders

ALLIUM CEPA
(Common Red Onion)

Characteristics
Primarily used for painful inflammation of upper air passages and hayfever.

Modalities
Worse:	Evening; warm room; odors.
Better:	Cold room (except cough); open air.

Clinical Picture
Eyes:	Profuse, non-irritating (unlike Euphrasia), watery discharge.
Nose:	Much sneezing with clear, copious dripping from nose that irritates the skin underneath.
Throat:	Raw throat and larynx.
Cough:	Cough triggered by tickling sensation in throat with aching in larynx. Holds larynx as it feels like it will tear with cough if not held. Cough can be triggered by inhalation of cold air.

Uses

1. Hayfever
2. Respiratory Infections
    b. Coughs and Colds
    d. Sore Throat

ANTIMONIUM TARTARICUM
(Tartrate of Antimony and Potash)

Characteristics
Confined largely to respiratory diseases; abundant bronchial secretions; great rattling of mucus with little expectoration. Drowsiness, debility and sweat. Heals bluish scars of acne or chickenpox.

Modalities
Worse: Evenings; lying down; damp, cold weather.
Better: Sitting erect; from eructation (belching) and expectoration.

Clinical Picture
Mental: Drowsy and despondent; fear of being alone; child will not be touched without whining.
Tongue: Coated, pasty, thick white.
Face: Pale; cold sweat; quivering chin and lower jaw.
Stomach: Thirst for cold water, nausea, retching and vomiting, especially after eating. Gagging or choking with cough (compare with Ipecac).
Lungs: Great rattling of mucus, but very little is expectorated. Often can only breathe with abdomen because of chest restriction. Asthma; bronchitis. Must sit up with cough.

Uses

1. Asthma
2. Chicken Pox

3. Collapse
4. Nausea and Vomiting

APIS MELLIFICA
(Honey Bee) (Apis)

Characteristics

Burning, sharp, stinging pains with pink swelling (like a bee sting) characterize this remedy. Swelling is both sudden and persistent, may be generalized or local in any tissue. Swellings may be very tender or sensitive to touch, as if bruised. Patient often tends to be fidgety.

Modalities

Worse: With warmth; pressure; afternoon (chill preceding fever), evening and night; lying down; becoming wet.

Better: By cold (room, air or application).

Clinical Picture

Eyes: Lids swollen, red, burning and stinging; some preference for right eye where face is involved.

Mouth: Red, shiny, puffy.

Stomach: Thirstless; sometimes craving for milk.

Abdomen: Can be extremely tender, sore, feeling of being bruised.

Urinary: Burning, pressing pain worse at the beginning of urination. Frequent, often constant painful urge to urinate. Child cries from agonizing pain before urinating. Cold helps. Bloody, cloudy, dark, milky, frothy or offensive urine.

Limbs: Hot, swollen, tender joint. Stinging pain.

Skin: Sudden appearance of pink or pale
swelling; may progress to purplish color if
deeper structure is involved. Severe,
sudden itching, stinging, burning sensation
and soreness. Feels better with cold
applications.

Uses

1. Abscesses
2. Fever
3. Headache
4. Injuries
   a. Bites, Stings and
      Puncture Wounds
   b. Sprains and
      Strains

5. Measles
6. Respiratory Infections
      d. Sore Throats
7. Skin Diseases
8. Styes
9. Urinary Problems

ARGENTUM NITRICUM
(Silver Nitrate)

Characteristics

Fears and anxiety accompany many conditions treated by this remedy. Though the person tends to crave sweets when ill, sweets make the condition worse. Problems tend to come on after intellectual work especially if accompanied by anticipation, fear or anxiety, such as feeling hurried about a deadline for work completion. Illness often occurs with unusual impulses such as a tendency to hurt one's self. Trembling, weakness and palpitations are common accompaniments of ailments. May feel clumsy when walking.

Modalities

Worse: Anticipation; fear; anxiety; sweets; intellectual work; heat; sleeping on right side.

Better: Fresh air (though headache sometimes worse in open air); pressure on painful region.

Clinical Picture

Mental: Anxiety, tends to hurry or be impulsive, particularly in anticipation of approaching deadline, whether deadline is real or magnified by the person's mind. Fear that has incurable disease, or will die when left alone. Easily angered or excited.

Vertigo: Dizzy from heights.

Head: Head feels large. Bones feel like they are separating. Boring pain left frontal eminence of forehead. Head feels better wrapped in a tight bandage. Headache triggered by unpleasant emotion. Can extend to the teeth.

Eyes: Inflammation of lids with discharge of pus. Light sensitivity.

Mouth: Sour taste in the mouth if headache extends to the teeth. Dry tongue with thirst. May be red down center with red tip, otherwise coated whitish gray. Can have fetid odor.

Throat: Red throat with splinter sensation on swallowing. Burning dryness with thick tenacious mucus in throat. May have ulceration and white patches.

Stomach: Craves sweets which aggravate. Nausea and vomiting of bile or sour fluid with headache.

Abdomen: Sensation of a lump. Gnawing pain which increases and decreases gradually and radiates in every direction. Feels worse with the least food. May find relief from bending double with fists in abdomen.

Rectum: Emotional diarrhea. Aggravation from drinking.

Stool: Shredded, mucus-filled stools, turning green like mashed spinach.

Lungs: Spasms of muscles make it difficult to breathe. Can't get breath once starts coughing. Can be triggered by laughing. Coughs up pus-filled mucus. Mucus in larynx can trigger cough, as can irritation under sternum. Hoarseness frequently accompanies the cough.

Uses

1. Asthma
2. Diarrhea
3. Headache

4. Respiratory Infections
    b. Coughs and Colds

ARNICA MONTANA
(Leopard's Bane, the Mountain Daisy) (Arnica)

Characteristics

Always the first remedy used internally for injury or over-exertion. Patient has feeling of bruised soreness with aching and pressing pains, hyper-acuteness of senses, fear of being approached or touched. Should be used externally over bruised area only if there is no broken skin. (Inflammation or irritation may result if used over broken skin.)

Modalities

Worse: Evenings and night; touch; pressure; physical exertion.

Better: Open air; lying down; with heat.

Clinical Picture

Mental: Fears touch or approach; feels bruised.

Head: Hot, with cold body.

Throat: Hoarseness from overuse of voice.

Limbs: Cannot walk or raise arms due to soreness.

Skin: Black and blue; bruises.

Uses

1. Abscesses and
      Inflammation
2. Bleeding
3. Collapse and Shock
4. Eye Disorders
5. Headache
6. Hoarseness
7. Injuries
   a. Wounds
   b. Bites, Stings, and
      Puncture Wounds
   c. Bruises
   d. Burns
   e. Sprains and Strains
8. Toothache

ARSENICUM ALBUM
(Arsenic Trioxide) (Arsenicum)

Characteristics

Characterized by burning pains relieved by heat; anxious; restless; weak and chilly with an air of fear and hopelessness. Tries to find relief in motion, but immediately feels weak with movement.

Restless. Feels cold. Complains of general weakness which is out of proportion to the apparent cause. Discharges are excoriating (burn the skin) and may smell like rotting flesh. Strong, intense thirst; drinks often but little at a time. Cold water disagrees.

Modalities

Worse:	Cold air, after midnight (particularly from 1:00 a.m. to 3:00 a.m.).
Better:	Warmth; open air, relieved by sweat. Hot drinks; lying down (but still restless).

Clinical Picture

Mental:	Fear with despair and restlessness.
Nose:	Thin, watery discharge that burns the skin around nose.
Throat:	Burning pain, relieved by hot drinks.
Stomach:	Aversion to sight or smell of food; burning pain.
Stool:	Diarrhea, with burning of rectum.
Lungs:	Unable to lie down, fears suffocation; cough worse after midnight.
Limbs:	Trembling, twitching.
Fever:	Fever worse between 12:00 a.m. to 2:00 a.m. Restlessness, yet feels weak.

Uses

1. Abdominal Pain
2. Asthma
3. Bleeding
4. Diarrhea
5. Fever
6. Hayfever
7. Indigestion
8. Nausea and Vomiting
9. Respiratory Infections
   b. Coughs and Colds
   d. Sore Throats
10. Toothache

BAPTISIA
(Wild Indigo)

Characteristics

Profound loss of energy with fever, influenza. Restless mind with lifeless body. Foul odors (breath, perspiration, stool, urine).

Modalities
Worse: On waking; walking; open air; cold wind.

Clinical Picture
Mental: Restless mind before delirium or with delirium in fever. Wandering mind that does not want to remain on one subject for any length of time. Sometimes head and limbs seem separate from body. Mistakes his own identity for that of two people. Can fall asleep while attempting to speak.

Head: Dull, heavy head; hard to hold up the head. Tight, drawn sensation, especially toward the back of the head and into the neck. Bruised sensation of brain and back of head. Frontal headache with pressure at root of nose.

Eyes: Very sensitive to light. Soreness of eyeballs, painful to read, hard to move.

Face: Hot, flushed face, dark red.

Mouth: Foul odor to breath. Papillae raised and project through white or yellow coating. Edges are deep red. Dry mouth with constant thirst for cold drinks. Flat, bitter taste in mouth.

Throat: Cannot swallow because of spasmodic pain; frequently can only succeed in swallowing

	water. Dark red. Tonsils swollen. Soreness.
Stomach:	Constant thirst for cold drinks.
Back:	Back and hips ache severely. Feels as if lying on hard board.
Limbs:	Tired and bruised, aches all over.
Sleep:	Constant desire to move, tries to find a softer spot in the bed. Tends to wake 2:00 a.m. to 3:00 a.m.

Uses

1. Fever
2. Respiratory Infections
   d. Sore Throats

BELLADONNA
(Deadly Nightshade)

Characteristics

Characterized by sudden, violent onset and rapid progression of symptoms.. High temperature; congestion; redness and throbbing with sweat only on covered parts. Predominantly right-sided. Hypersensitivity to all sensations with heightened nervous excitability that can cause acute delirium. Twitching of muscles and spasms of internal organs with sensations of constriction or fullness. Pains are usually throbbing and stabbing, appear suddenly and then disappear and reappear again.

Modalities

Worse: Touch; motion; cold (particularly drafts); lying down; 3:00 p.m. to midnight.

Better: Heat; sitting still and upright; covering up.

Clinical Picture

Mental: Acuteness of all senses; tends toward delirium; restless, especially while sleeping; may cry out during sleep because of nightmares.

Head: Throbbing pain with sensation of fullness, especially in forehead.

Face: Red, especially cheeks; hot; dry.

Eyes: Pupils dilated; eyes feel swollen; glassy-eyed.

Ears: Tearing pain.

Tongue: Red on edges, white with red spots (strawberry looking).

Throat: Dry, red, constricted, painful swelling; glands swollen and tender.

Stomach: No appetite; either extreme thirst or aversion to liquids.

Abdomen: Pain, much worse with jarring, better bending forward.

Female: Bearing down pains, worse lying down, better by standing (opposite of Sepia). Early menstruation of profuse, bright red blood. If flow is darker, it is offensive in odor. Paroxysmal (come and go suddenly) cutting pains in a horizontal direction. If there is inflammation of an ovary, right side is more often affected.

Lungs: Tickling, short, dry cough; worse at night. Larynx very painful.

Fever: Dry, hot, "burns" your hand; perspiration on covered parts.

Uses

1. Abdominal Pain
2. Bleeding
3. Ear problems
4. Fever
5. Headache
6. Measles
7. Menstrual Problems
8. Mumps
9. Respiratory Infections
   b. Coughs and Colds
   d. Sore Throats
10. Toothache

BORAX
(Sodium Borate)

Characteristics

Poor nutritional status precipitates many of the problems for which Borax is indicated in treatment. Tendency to ulceration of shriveled, unhealthy mucous membranes. Dread of downward motion. Helpful in thrush and yeast infections.

Modalities

Worse: Downward motion (laying sleeping child down or carrying child downstairs, for example). Noise.

Clinical Picture

Mental: Great anxiety from downward motion. Child tolerates motion as long as it is not downward. Baby wakes and cries out when attempting to lay the child down. Startles from least noise. Infant screams before urination in fearful anticipation of pain that will come. Irritable before stool, better after. Fusses before nursing and refuses, though nurses well as soon as the mouth is moistened.

Eyes: Gummy, crusty lids.

Ear: Swollen, hot ear like Belladonna, Pulsatilla, Chamomilla.

Nose: Ulceration from acrid discharge that is clear, copious, like egg-white, feels hot like other secretions, and may be gummy and crusty eye secretions.

Face: Pale.

Mouth:	Ulcerations; canker sores. Mouth feels very hot to touch (such as infant's mouth when nursing). Ulcers start as small, red fluid-filled vesicles. Ulcers have sensation as if burnt and are painful to the least touch. Pain with contact of acidic and salty foods. Roof of mouth shriveled. Dry, cracked tongue.
Urine:	Hot, acrid urine with urgency. Soreness in urethra on touch.
Female:	Thrush. Thick, corrosive, starch-like discharge. Stinging, swollen sensation in clitoris. Sensation of burning in vagina.
Rectum:	Diarrhea.
Stool:	Green with mucus.
Skin:	Unhealthy; festers easily; won't heal. Vesicular eruption.

Uses

1. Travel Sickness
2. Vaginitis

BRYONIA ALBA
(Bryonia) (Wild Hops)

Characteristics

The hallmark of Bryonia is aggravation from motion; the least change of position in some distant part aggravates the pain. Dryness with great thirst for large quantities at long intervals.

Typical Bryonia patient is irritable, inclined to be vehement, and has angry outbursts when disturbed. All internal surfaces feel dry from mouth to joints, lungs, abdomen and pelvic area. Symptoms usually develop slowly (contrast with Aconite, Belladonna). Called the "sleeping bear" remedy. Bryonia is like the bear which is often gentle and playful, but can be irritable or violent if disturbed.

Modalities

Worse: Motion; inhalation; touch; sitting up; warmth; cold, dry wind; eating.

Better: Lying on painful side; absolute rest; cold; eating cold things; firm pressure.

Clinical Picture

Mind: Irritable; doesn't want to be bothered; desires seclusion in dark room.

Head: Bursting, splitting headaches as if everything pressed out. Worse on motion.

Nose: Dry.

Mouth: Lips parched, dry, cracked; bitter taste.

Tongue: White coating.

Stomach: Nausea and faintness upon rising; vomiting of bile and water immediately after eating; warm drinks are vomited. Worse with the slightest movement.

Abdomen: Sensitive to touch.

Stool: Constipated; stools dry, as if burnt.

Female: Marked pain in right ovary, aggravated by touch, extending down to the thighs. Can have profuse, dark flow or suppression of flow.

Lungs: Dry, hacking cough, especially at night; must sit up when coughing.

Uses

1. Abdominal Pain
2. Bleeding
3. Diarrhea
4. Fever
5. Headache
6. Indigestion
7. Injuries
    e. Sprains and Strains

8. Measles
9. Menstrual Problems
10. Nausea and Vomiting
11. Respiratory Infections
    b. Coughs and Colds
    d. Sore Throats
12. Travel Sickness

CALCAREA CARBONICUM
(Calcium Carbonate, Impure) (Calcarea Ostrearum)

Characteristics

Decreased energy and slowness. Sensitive to cold, feels like a draft of air goes right through the body. Body feels cold to touch as well as having an internal sensation of coldness. May feel cold only in spots. May perspire on isolated areas such as the scalp only, or the upper chest only. Tends to feel better generally when constipated. Ailments tend to come on from exposure to cold, from fears or from over consumption of calcium-containing foods such as dairy products. Tends to have swollen glands, especially the back of the neck.

Modalities

Worse: Cold in all forms: weather, cold drinks or cool baths. Exertion: physical or mental.
Better: Dry weather.

Clinical Picture

Mental: Apprehensive, especially toward evening.
Head: Perspiration on scalp only (Silica tends to involve the entire head and often the neck). Headache is worse at change of weather, from motion, in the open air and from stooping. Head and face feel hot during headache or from mental exertion. Feels better lying still. Pain can radiate from the forehead to the nose, from the temples to the jaws or from the muscles of the back of the neck to the base of the skull. Dizziness and nausea often present with headache.
Eyes: Sensitive to light, lachrymation.

Ears:	Rupture is common with fatty-looking bland discharge (like chewed up paper). May have fluid-filled vesicle or polyps on the eardrum. Swollen glands, slow to resolve, especially on the back of the neck. Noises in the ears.
Nose:	Dry by day, runny at night. Stopped up in warm air or out-of-doors. Runny in cold air. Wings of nose may be thickened and ulcerated. Offensive odor of manure, rotten eggs, or gunpowder with thick, yellow pus stopping up the nose.
Mouth:	Painless hoarseness, hardly audible voice, worse in the morning and better by hawking. Tip of tongue sore; acid saliva; bad taste.
Teeth:	Sensitive to chewing. Pain worse at night. Subject to slow tooth eruption or to rapid decay.
Throat:	Achiness in morning, worse with swallowing and may extend down the esophagus to the stomach on swallowing. Contracted sensation in the throat. Often also has chronic swelling of tonsils.
Stomach:	Vomiting, especially right after taking milk. Ravenous appetite and thirst. May crave or be averse to milk, but milk disagrees. Craves eggs. Feels sick if eats fat when ill.
Rectum:	Summer diarrhea, especially after milk. Worse evening.
Stool:	Often green, watery, sour, with undigested food. Milk may pass undigested.
Female:	Too frequent and profuse menstrual flow accompanied by pain in the breasts before menses and head sweat with cold feet.

Emotional stress increases the flow. Leucorrhea, when present, is profuse, burning, itching, and may be milky or yellow and thick. Especially indicated for discharges occurring in infants or before puberty.

Lungs: Cough dry at night, becoming loose in the morning. Notices shortness of breath, palpitations and rush of blood to the chest on exertion. May have partial sweat, especially on the upper chest. Sore to touch, especially under the collarbone. Right lung tends to be affected more often than left. Coughs up yellow, green expectoration, sometimes with blood in it.

Uses

1. Diarrhea
2. Ear Problems
3. Headache
4. Hoarseness
5. Menstrual Problems
6. Nausea and Vomiting

7. Respiratory Infections
    b. Coughs and Colds
    c. Sinus Infections
    d. Sore Throats
8. Toothache
9. Vaginitis

CALCAREA PHOSPHORICUM
(Calcium Phosphate)

Characteristics

Picture of whining, teething infants accompanied by discharges, such as diarrhea or respiratory cleansing. Respiratory symptoms often come up in spring with change to wet, cold weather. Symptoms may come on with growth spurts.

Modalities

Worse:	Damp, cold weather.
Better:	Warm, dry weather.

Clinical Picture

Mental:	Peevish; fretful; whiny.
Head:	Headache worse moving, worse stooping or change of position, better open air or lying still.
Nose:	Drains in cold room; stuffed up in warm room or out-of-doors. Sneezing with flow of mucus from nose and increased saliva (may have acid taste).
Teeth:	Pain, worse warm or cold things in mouth.
Stomach:	Infant wants to nurse constantly. Colic.
Rectum:	Diarrhea after sharp pain. Green, loose and slimy stools though may also be hot and watery.
Female:	Weak, empty sinking feeling in lower abdomen. Cream-like discharge or discharge like egg-white. Burning in vagina with pain in bladder and uterus. Burning may extend up into chest. Menses often too early, too long-lasting, and profuse in slender women prone to spells of

low energy. Often indicated in painful menses around puberty. Labor-like pains before and during flow. Uterine spasms after urination or bowel movements. Sore breasts during pregnancy.

Lungs: Tickling cough; yellow phlegm; worse in morning. Breath short, seems difficult. Hoarseness. Tends to clear throat.

Limbs: Achiness ("growing pains").

Uses

1. Asthma
2. Dentition (teething)
3. Diarrhea
4. Headache

5. Menstrual Problems
6. Respiratory Infections
      b. Colds and Coughs
7. Vaginitis

CALENDULA OFFICINALIS
(Marigold) (Calendula)

Characteristics

Used externally as ointment or lotion (mother tincture diluted with water) for injuries involving cutting, tearing or other mechanical forms of injury; damage to surface of skin, exposing underlying living tissue. Calendula provides protection against infection and promotes healing.

Dosage and Administration

Always use externally. Lotion is prepared by diluting one teaspoon Calendula mother tincture to one cup water. Lotion is useful when short-term soaking is indicated; ointment should be used for longer applications (overnight).

Uses

1. Eye Disorders
2. Injuries
       a. Wounds
             1. Incised
             2. Lacerated
       b. Bites, Scratches and Puncture Wounds
       c. Bruises
       d. Burns

CANTHARIS VESICATOR
(Spanish fly) (Cantharis)

Characteristics

Used for burns or scalds. Excessive burning pains (eyes, mouth, throat, stomach, intestinal tract); frequent urge to urinate with burning, passing a few drops of urine at a time; stringy, tenacious discharges from mucus membranes. Vesicles or blisters full of yellowish fluid quickly becoming filled with pus, burning like fire. Anxious restlessness ending in rage.

Modalities

Worse: Night; cold; pressure; coffee.
Better: Lying down.

Clinical Picture

Throat: Burning in mouth and throat; difficult to swallow liquids.

Stomach: Burning sensation of esophagus and stomach. Burning thirst, with aversion to all fluids.

Urinary: Intolerable urge to urinate with cutting pain extending to urethra. Burns before, during or after urination. Pain in bladder at beginning of urination, extending to kidneys. May urinate drop by drop, each drop having agonizing pain. Burning is relieved by heat. Urine acrid, bloody, cloudy, dark or red. Can have sediment or pus.

Skin: Burns with blisters. Vesicles that burn and itch. Sunburn.

Uses

1. Injuries
        b. Bites, Stings and Puncture Wounds
        d. Burns
2. Respiratory Infections
        d. Sore Throats
3. Urinary Problems

CARBO VEGETABILIS
(Vegetable Charcoal) (Carbo Vegetabilis)

Characteristics

Patient exhibits mental and physical sluggishness and symptoms come on slowly. Generalized weakness of all functions, especially digestion. Often overweight, torpid, lazy. Complaints of coldness (general or local). Symptoms may date to inadequate recovery from previous exhausting disease. Pains usually described as burning, pressing pains. Must have fresh air; wishes to be fanned. Digestive problems such as belching often accompany any illness for which Carbo Vegetabilis is useful.

Modalities

Worse: Morning and evening; exertion; cold; tight clothes at abdomen.

Better: Being fanned; passing gas; rest.

Clinical Picture

Head: Aches from overindulgence.

Face: Puffy, gray-blue; pale.

Nose: Bleeds daily.

Stomach: Belching; heaviness; fullness. "Contraction-like" pain extending to chest, with distention of abdomen. The abdomen is distended with flatulent colic. Simplest food disagrees. Aversion to milk, meats and fatty foods.

Lungs: Wheezing in old people. Asthma comes on after overeating and may be accompanied by belching and fullness in stomach.

Female: Depressed with menses. Strong odor to flow. Feeling of weight in uterus and right ovary. Dragging sensation in abdomen and small of back. Burning, thin discharge with

sore ulcerations.   Itching discharge.
Burning across sacrum and deep in pelvis
with discharge.   Pains increase and
decrease.

Uses

1. Asthma
2. Bleeding
3. Collapse and Shock
4. Hoarseness
5. Indigestion

6. Menstrual Problems
7. Respiratory Infections
   b. Coughs and Colds
8. Vaginitis

CHAMOMILLA
(German Chamomile)

Characteristics

Chief symptoms are emotional, which usually lead to body disturbances. Frequently found in children who are restless, irritable, whining and colicky. Sensitive, especially to pain. Thirsty, hot, numb sensation with unbearable pains. (Mental calmness, constipation rule against Chamomilla.) Useful for prolonged side effects of novocaine and may be useful to decrease cravings or addiction to cocaine and other narcotics.

Modalities

Worse: Heat; anger; night; with wind.
Better: Being carried; warm, wet weather.

Clinical Picture

Mental: Cross, nothing satisfies child except being carried. Soothing objects demanded, yet refused or thrown when offered.
Ears: Feel hot; pain driving patient frantic.
Teeth: Teething children who are cross and complaining; toothache after warm drinks, relieved by cold drinks or ice.
Face: Hot with redness often only on one side.
Tongue: Yellow coat.
Stomach: Acid; belching.
Abdomen: Colic; gas after anger. Hot perspiration.
Stool: Hot, green, watery, looks like chopped eggs and spinach.

Uses

1. Abdominal Pain
2. Dentition (teething)
3. Diarrhea
4. Ear Problems
5. Indigestion
6. Nausea and Vomiting
7. Toothache

CHINA (CINCHONA OFFICINALIS)
(Quinine) (Peruvian Bark)

Characteristics

Effects of loss of bodily fluids from such conditions as hemorrhage (including delivery of babies), prolonged nursing, sweating or diarrhea. Rapid, general weakness with tendency to perspire from least exertion of movement as well as during sleep. Desires to fan self. Weight loss.

Modalities

Worse:	After loss of fluids. Touch aggravates (though rubbing helps). Cold drafts (pain).
Better:	Rubbing.

Clinical Picture

Mind:	May have delirium with fever.
Head:	Headache from loss of fluids with heaviness and faintness.
Face:	Red.
Ear:	Buzzing in ears. Sounds seem as if they are heard from great distance.
Mouth:	Everything tastes bitter.
Stomach:	Thirstless, even with fever, until perspiring, then intense thirst. Hunger, but feels full easily. Vomiting, if present, tends to be of acidic, slimy matter, water or food. Vomiting is associated with accumulation of water in the mouth.
Rectum:	Painless diarrhea, worse at night and after eating (podophyllum usually worse during the day). Tends to occur in hot weather, especially after eating fruit.
Stool:	Yellow, brown, watery stool, often with undigested food.

Fever: No thirst during chill or long heat that follows. Wants heat source during chill, but does not feel better when provided. Desires to uncover during heat. Following long heat there is profuse sweating with intense thirst. Can have periodic fever, such as every two, or less commonly, every three days.

Uses

1. Diarrhea
2. Fever
3. Nausea and Vomiting

COCCULUS INDICUS
(Indian Cockle)

Characteristics

Travel sickness. Weakness from nausea, vertigo, or loss of sleep. Irritable and hypersensitive to pain. Coldness of limbs. Ill effects of anger and grief.

Modalities

Worse: Motion of airplanes, boats and cars. Lack of sleep. From tobacco smoke. Noise.

Better: With warmth. Lying quietly.

Clinical Picture

Stomach: Nausea with vertigo and sick headache from riding in airplanes, boats and cars. Better with warmth. Aversion to food, even the smell of food. Tense feeling below the stomach as if the waist was constricted by a tight band.

Abdomen: Colic with rectal flatus. Colic from nervousness and from menses. The bowels feel as if the intestines were being pinched between sharp stones, with pain so great that fainting and vomiting may follow. Cutting and burning pain as from an incarcerated hernia, worse after rising from sitting.

Stool: Thin, yellowish, painless stools only in the daytime. Diarrhea from riding in the car, even the shortest distance. Diarrhea with the sensation of sharp stones rubbing together in the abdomen. Intense rectal pain after passing the stool, pain which may lead to fainting.

Uses

1. Abdominal Pain
2. Diarrhea
3. Nausea and Vomiting
4. Travel Sickness

COFFEA CRUDA
(Unroasted Coffee)

Characteristics

Increased activity of the nerves and senses. Onset of illness may be from teething, overwork, too much stimulating food or drink, and from emotional surprises (especially pleasant surprises). Over-excited and talkative. Children at times cannot bear to be carried about (like Chamomilla). Violent throbbing toothache.

Modalities

Worse: From cold, except for toothaches which cold relieves. Noise.

Better: With heat, except for toothaches.

Clinical Picture

Mind: Easily excited and irritated. Tossing about with anguish. Intolerant to all physical and emotional pain.

Mouth: Teething. Toothaches with excessive pain, which are better holding cold water or ice in the mouth. The toothache returns as the mouth warms up again. Worse from warm drinks and chewing.

Sleep: Mental activity prevents sleep. Restless and wakeful. Imperfect sleep with eyes half-open.

Uses

1. Dentition (teething)
2. Toothache

COLCHICUM AUTUMNALE
(Meadow Saffron)

Characteristics

Nausea, especially in pregnancy. Hypersensitive to odors. Hunger and weakness from vomiting. Dysentery and diarrhea in the hot, humid weather of autumn. Gout.

Modalities

Worse: From motion and movement (Bryonia). From cold (opposite of Bryonia). Strong odors of food. From sunset until sunrise.

Better: With warmth. Stooping or bending double (as in curling up in a ball, with knees drawn to the chest). Better at daybreak.

Clinical Picture

Mind: Suffering seems intolerable; all external impressions of light, noise and strong odors will disturb their temper.

Stomach: Nausea, especially in the first months of pregnancy, when finding food offensive. Disgust at the thought, sight or smell of food. All attempts to eat cause violent nausea and vomiting. The smell of food can create intense nausea which leads to fainting. Violent retching. Better when curled up in a ball.

Stools: Extremely painful stools with violent urging. Diarrhea in the hot, humid weather.

Limbs: Gout, cannot bear to have the limb touched or moved. Stubbing the toe causes great pain. Acute rheumatism.

Uses

1. Diarrhea
2. Nausea and Vomiting

COLOCYNTHIS
(Bitter Cucumber)

Characteristics

Ill effects of suppressed anger. Often for women with sedentary habits and heavy build. Severe, tearing pains relieved by pressure; cramping pains especially in abdomen causing patient to double over. Useful for menstrual cramps. Often indicated in changing seasons, when air is cold but sun still heats the body.

Modalities

Worse: Suppressed emotion; least amount of food.
Better: Pressure; heat; bending over; escape of gas; passing stool.

Clinical Picture

Mind: Irritable when pains come.
Abdomen: Sensation as if the intestines were being pinched between sharp stones, with pain so great that fainting and vomiting may follow. Abdomen feels like it will burst; bruised feeling; soreness around navel; worse with least amount of food. Draws knees to chest for relief.
Stomach: Nausea and vomiting with pains.
Stools: Jelly-like.
Female: Gripping ovarian pain, causing to bend double to seek relief. Also relieved by heat and strong pressure. Can be particularly triggered following violent emotion.
Limbs: Pains; contractions of hips and legs; burning; sciatica.

Uses

1. Abdominal Pain
2. Diarrhea
3. Headache
4. Indigestion
5. Menstrual Problems
6. Nausea and Vomiting

CUPRUM
(The Metal, Copper)

Characteristics
Coughs and cramps. Symptoms can be intense and violent; spasmodic pains that start and end suddenly. There are no passive symptoms with this remedy. All symptoms are improved by cold drinks. Mental and physical exhaustion from loss of sleep and over-exertion of the mind.

Modalities
Worse: At night; from touch or pressure.
Better: On drinking cold water, especially for cough and vomiting.

Clinical Picture
Mouth: Strong metallic taste (like Mercurius and Rhus Toxicodendron). Desires cold food and drink.
Stomach: Nausea. Stomach cramps that come and go, with nausea and vomiting. Improves with drinking cold water. Vomiting with cough.
Abdomen: Violent, contracted spasms of the abdomen and upper and lower limbs, with piercing, distressing screams. Colic which is violent and intermittent. Most distressing after-pains from childbirth, particularly in women who have borne many children.
Rectum: Violent diarrhea with intense abdominal cramps. Weakness from stool, with restlessness and tossing about.
Lungs: Cough in spasms, worse inhaling cool air. Whooping cough. Spasm and constriction of chest.

Limbs: Muscle spasms, usually beginning in toes
            and fingers and then spreading. Cramps in
            the calves, contracted like knots. Coldness
            of feet.

Uses

1. Abdominal Pain
2. Diarrhea
3. Nausea and Vomiting
4. Respiratory Infections
        b. Coughs and Colds

DROSERA
(Sundew)

Characteristics
Chiefly confined to use in respiratory ailments for the purposes of this book.

Clinical Picture
Lungs: Barking cough. Cannot recover breathing because of high frequency of coughing. Cannot cough deep enough to obtain relief. After midnight (or early evening and then again after midnight). Vomiting or retching if not able to raise mucus.

Uses

1. Respiratory Infections
   a. Croup
   b. Coughs and Colds

DULCAMARA
(Bitter Sweet)

Characteristics
Often called the "wet remedy". Indicated for troubles which result from getting wet and chilled. Ailments made worse in damp, cold weather, especially at close of summer when warm days suddenly change to cold nights. Ill effects of sitting on cold, damp ground or getting chilled on a rainy day.

Modalities
Worse: Night; cold in general; damp, rainy weather.
Better: Moving around; external warmth.

Clinical Picture
Nose: Stuffy in cold dampness; alternating blocked and profuse discharge.
Throat: Thirst.
Abdomen: Gripping pains around navel.
Stools: Green, watery, especially at night.
Lungs: Loose cough.
Feet: Very cold.

Uses

1. Hayfever
2. Respiratory Infections
    b. Coughs and Colds

EQUISETUM HYEMALE
(Scouring-rush)

Characteristics
   Remedy used principally for urinary complaints.

Modalities
   Worse: Pressing; movement.

Clinical Picture
   Urinary: Constant desire to urinate as if bladder is
                 full. Urination does not relieve the urge.
                 Tender   bladder,   worse   pressure.
                 Involuntary urination, dribbling, especially
                 at night. Pain in right kidney. Testicles
                 may ache. Heaviness and aching in bladder
                 which remains after urination. Prickling,
                 cutting pain in urethra after urination.
                 Burning in urethra during or after urination.
                 Mucus in urine (different from Cantharis).

Uses

1. Urinary Problems

EUPATORIUM PERFOLIATUM
(Thoroughwort)

Characteristics

Good remedy for many cases of influenza. Achiness all through body impels to change position without relief. May have periodicity such as chill one morning, then evening the next day.

Modalities

Worse: Lying left side.

Better: Perspiration relieves all symptoms except headache. Cough better on hands and knees.

Clinical Picture

Head: Feels sore internally. Eyeballs sore with headache. Head feels better on first going outside.

Lungs: Extreme soreness along trachea (windpipe). May hold chest with hands on coughing. Is worse on left side but better getting on hands and knees. Worse 2:00 a.m. to 4:00 a.m. Cough excited by tickling in chest. Chest is sore during inspiration. Hoarseness in morning.

Limbs: Aching in limbs, worse with high fever, better with perspiration. Feels impelled to move, but movement does not relieve.

Chill: Begins often 7:00 a.m. to 9:00 a.m. with headache preceding and insatiable thirst. This thirst rarely continues into the fever. Chill generally begins in the small of the back. May be periodic, first one morning, then again the next evening.

Uses

1. Fever
2. Respiratory Infections
        b. Coughs and Colds

EUPHRASIA OFFICINALIS
(Eyebright)

Characteristics
Particularly useful for its action on mucus membranes of eyes and nose.

Modalities
Worse:	Light; warmth; indoors.
Better:	Dark.

Clinical Picture
Eyes:	Profuse tearing, burning the cheeks. Eyes red, puffy; may have ulceration. Film may form; blurred vision relieved by wiping eyes. Not relieved by warm water (unlike Arsenicum Album or Rhus Toxicodendron). May have stinging, shooting pains.
Nose:	Bland non-irritating drainage in contrast to eyes.
Cough:	Gags when clearing throat in morning because of profuse drainage.

Uses

1. Hayfever

FERRUM PHOSPHORICUM
(Iron Phosphate) (Ferrum Phos)

Characteristics

Indicated in ailments of generalized inflammation, characterized by pain, fever, redness and a quickened pulse. Used for fevers and inflammation before pus accumulates. Can substitute for Aconite, but actually stands midway between Aconite and Gelsemium in its staging of inflammation, fever and weakness.

Modalities
Worse:	Motion; night.
Better:	Cold applications.

Clinical Picture
Head:	Aching with rush of blood; headache from heat of sun.
Eyes:	Red; burning; sore; sensation of grain of sand under lid.
Ears:	First stage of earache with tension, throbbing and heat.
Nose:	Bleeding, especially in children.
Face:	Flushed.
Tongue:	Clean and reddened.
Throat:	Sore; dry; red; inflamed; painful; no pus yet.
Urinary:	Frequent urge to urinate with pain from lower bladder to tip of urethra. Feels urge to urinate immediately in order to relieve the pain. Tends to be worse during the day and worse standing. Better lying down.
Lungs:	First stages of cough.
Skin:	Measles and scarlet fever (first stage of fever).

Uses

1. Abdominal Pain
2. Abscesses and
      Inflammation
3. Bleeding
4. Chicken Pox
5. Ear Problems
6. Fever
7. Headache
8. Hoarseness
9. Measles
10. Mumps
11. Respiratory Infections
      b. Coughs and Colds
      d. Sore Throats
12. Styes
13. Toothache
14. Urinary Problems

GELSEMIUM SEMPERVIRENS
(Yellow Jasmine) (Gelsemium)

Characteristics

"The great paralyzer," drowsiness, grogginess, trembling, listlessness, dullness, heaviness. Problems often brought on by grief, bad news or anticipation. Muscular weakness. Patient has no appetite or thirst. Symptoms have a slow onset; preceded by weakness, languor and desire to lie down. Symptoms may be brought on by warm, humid weather. Upon waking, there is trembling and a sense of heaviness. Frequently an influenza remedy.

Modalities

Worse: Damp weather; before storms; bad news; thinking about ailment; 10:00 a.m.

Better: Bending forward; urinating; perspiration; open air.

Clinical Picture

Head: Dull, heavy ache; muscle soreness in neck and shoulders. Dizziness when carried or needs to hang onto furniture to support self; headache begins in nape of neck and settles over the eyes. Usually worse in early morning.

Eyes: Eyelids heavy.

Nose: Sneezing, running, fullness and pain at root of nose. Nostrils and wings of nose raw and sore; sneezing in morning.

Tongue: Thick, yellowish coating; trembling.

Throat: Difficulty swallowing; sore, rough, burning throat; pain in ears when swallowing.

Stomach: Absence of hunger or thirst.

Stool:	Cream-colored or tea-green-colored diarrhea.
Lungs:	Dry, sore cough with teasing, tickling sensation and little expectoration. May sound croupy.
Back:	Aching with ascending chill.
Skin:	Measles—before rash, helps bring rash out. Itching prevents sleep.
Fever:	Intermittent with heat; nervous, restless, yet too weak to move. Child may ask to be moved. Red faced. Thirstless. Perspiration relieves symptoms.

Uses

1. Diarrhea
2. Fever
3. Hayfever
4. Headache
5. Hoarseness

6. Measles
7. Respiratory Infections
    b. Coughs and Colds
    d. Sore Throats

HELONIAS DIOICA
(Unicorn Plant) (Helonias)

Characteristics
Remedy for vaginitis, especially during pregnancy. Profound depression often accompanies uterine complaints.

Modalities
Worse: Exertion, especially lifting or walking.

Clinical Picture
Mental: Sadness, often profound.
Mouth: Can have increase in saliva.
Urinary: Burning, scalding with urination. Frequent urging. Burning sensation in kidneys.
Female: Heaviness and soreness of lower pelvis with constant voluminous discharge, usually white, like sour, curdled milk though may be dark and coagulated if blood is present. Discharge causes itching and may produce redness, swelling or ulceration of vulva. Discharge and heavy, sore sensation aggravated by exertion, especially lifting.
Back: Soreness in uterus may extend to small of back.

Uses

1. Vaginitis

HEPAR SULPHURIS CALCAREUM
(Sulphate of Lime and Hahnemann's Calcium Sulphide)
(Hepar Sulph)

Characteristics

Often peevish, angry at slightest provocation and hypochondriacal. Very sensitive to cold drafts, tending to catch cold. Infected yellow or green discharges freely flow from mucous membranes.

Modalities

Worse:	Dry, cold winds; draft; lying on right side.
Better:	Damp weather; warmth; after eating.

Clinical Picture

Head:	Boring, aching pain at root of nose and forehead above eyes, especially when waking from sleep. Worse motion, stooping, moving eyes. Better warmth.
Ears:	Throbbing, buzzing. Useful to help eliminate fluid behind ear drum.
Nose:	Soreness of nostrils; sneezes in cold winds; yellow or green drainage.
Face:	Yellowish complexion. Pains of bones on parts being touched. Drawing, tearing pains extend to ears or temples.
Teeth:	Tender abscess of gum especially with inflammation and tenderness where tooth meets gum or over erupting tooth, especially wisdom tooth.
Neck:	Swollen, tender lymph glands.
Throat:	Feels as though plug or splinter is lodged when swallowing. Pain from throat to ear when swallowing. Throat pain; sensitive to draft on neck.

Abdomen: Pain in upper right side under ribs; worse with cough or breathing.

Lungs: Choking, croupy, strangulating cough. Worse being uncovered or eating cold food. Wheezing. Loose cough.

Skin: Unhealthy skin that forms ulcer from small scratches.

Uses

1. Abscesses and
    Inflammation
2. Ear Problems
3. Hoarseness
4. Respiratory Infections
    a. Croup
    b. Coughs and Colds
    c. Sinus Infections
    d. Sore Throats
5. Styes
6. Toothache

HYPERICUM PERFOLIATUM
(St. John's Wort) (Hypericum)

Characteristics

Indicated if pain of injury radiates from initial site toward center of body. Very useful to relieve pain; helps heal injuries to nerve-rich areas (toes, fingertips, gums). Hypericum is the Arnica of the spinal column. Falls on or blows to the spine, particularly the tailbone (coccyx), respond to Hypericum. Hypericum ointment or lotion may be used on some skin wounds, particularly those that appear infected and where pain is associated with the area of injury.

Uses

1. Eye Disorders
2. Injuries
     a. Wounds
          1. Incised Wounds
          2. Lacerated Wounds
          3. Scratches and Abrasions
     b. Bites, Stings and Puncture Wounds
     c. Bruises
     d. Burns

IGNATIA AMARA
(St. Ignatius' Bean) (Ignatia)

Characteristics
Emotional state is of quickly alternating moods, extreme nervousness with trembling inside. Especially suited for nervous, sensitive, highly conscientious, excitable (sadness and weeping) people with gentle dispositions. A remedy of erratic, contradictory, paradoxical symptoms. Condition may arise after disappointment or from grief.

Modalities
Worse: Morning. Coffee. External warmth.
Better: Change of position. Hard pressure.

Clinical Picture
Head: Congestion after anger or grief; worse from strong odors. Pain is in one spot as if nail were driven through head. Brought on by irksome work. Better after urination.

Throat: Feeling as if lump were in throat. Difficulty swallowing. Lump sensation worse when not swallowing. Yellowish-white, small ulcers.

Stomach: Sinking, empty feeling; worse with deep breath. Vomiting with headaches.

Rectum: Diarrhea from fright. Stabbing pains up rectum. Itching.

Female: Menses dark, frequent, and with large amount of flow. Labor-like pains better by pressure, by lying on back, and by change of position. Corrosive, pus-filled discharge preceded by spasms of the uterus.

Lungs: Hollow, spasmodic cough.   Sighing.
             Sensation of feather in throat triggers cough
             and becomes worse with coughing.
Fever: Thirst during the chill. Warmth or covering
             relieves chill. (Nux Vomica not relieved
             this way; Arsenicum Album and Rhus
             Toxicodendron chills are relieved by
             warmth.)

Uses

1. Headache   5. Travel Sickness
2. Indigestion   6. Vaginitis
3. Menstrual Problems
4. Respiratory Infection
      d. Sore Throats

IPECACUANHA
(Ipecac Root) (Ipecac)

Characteristics

Most indicated for complaints of persistent nausea not relieved by vomiting; ailments caused by eating rich or indigestible foods such as ice cream, sweets (compare with Nux Vomica, Pulsatilla). Useful to stop bleeding if blood is bright red.

Modalities

Worse: Warm, moist weather. Lying down.

Clinical Picture

Mental: Easily irritated, child cries or screams continuously, wanting something but not certain what they desire.

Eyes: Blue rings around eyes.

Tongue: Clean.

Throat: Thirstless.

Stomach: Constant nausea and vomiting.

Abdomen: Flatulent; clutching pain around navel.

Lungs: Asthma returning periodically. Cough incessant with each breath; feels full of mucus but nothing comes up. Vomits during asthma.

Stool: Greenish diarrhea, consistency of frothy molasses.

Uses

1. Abdominal Pain
2. Asthma
3. Bleeding
4. Diarrhea
5. Hoarseness
6. Indigestion
7. Nausea and Vomiting

IRIS VERSICOLOR
(Blue Flag Plant) (Iris)

Characteristics

Headache remedy, especially for those that come on after a letdown following a period of stress, such as a weekend after a week of study or stressful work. Often preceded by visual symptoms and burning gastric distress.

Modalities

Better: Cold drinks.

Clinical Picture

Head: Frontal headache or periodic migraine, right more often than left. Brought on by letdown after stress. Can come periodically, such as every weekend after a letdown following study or work.

Eyes: Cloudy vision before headache. Can have temporary blindness with headache.

Mouth: Feels greasy and scalded. Much ropy saliva and sweet taste.

Stomach: Burning, acidic vomiting with headache. Burning of entire digestive tract. Some relief with cold drinks. Vomiting often starts in early morning, 2:00 a.m. to 3:00 a.m.

Stool: Burning, watery stools.

Uses

1. Headache

KALI BICHROMICUM
(Potassium Bichromate)

Characteristics
Mucus membranes. Tough, stringy, viscid secretions, sometimes forming thick, yellow-green mucus. Sinus infections. Fat, chubby babies predisposed to colds.

Modalities
Worse: Cold; beer; morning; undressing.
Better: Heat.

Clinical Picture
Nose: Thick, ropy, yellow-green mucus, may be bloody, can form crusts in the nose. Pressure and pain at the root of the nose and cheekbones. Frontal and maxillary sinusitis. Snuffles of children. Violent sneezing. Obstruction of the nose.

Mouth: Dry; viscid saliva.

Throat: Swollen, red, dry with unquenchable thirst. Ulceration on the tonsils. Swollen glands. Stringy mucus.

Lungs: Profuse, yellow expectoration which is sticky, stringy. Voice hoarse. Metallic cough. Croup. Wakes from sleep because of choking.

Uses

1. Asthma
2. Headache
3. Respiratory Infections
       a. Croup
       c. Sinus Infections

KALI CARBONICUM
(Potassium Carbonate)

Characteristics

Mucus membranes: digestive and respiratory. Very tired, anemic individual. Flabby tissues, which may be swollen. Sweat, backache, weakness. Many conditions have an aggravation at 2:00 a.m. to 4:00 a.m. Often stays immobile when ill.

Modalities

Worse: Cold weather; between 2:00 a.m. to 4:00 a.m.

Better: During the day. Sitting down. Bending forward. Warmth.

Clinical Picture

Mental: Very irritable. Hypersensitive to pain. Despondent.

Eyes: Swollen above upper lids.

Nose: Stuffs up in a warm room. Thick, yellow discharge; forms crusts. Soreness.

Stomach: Anxiety felt in stomach. Acidic, upset stomach; nausea which is better while lying down. Craves sweets. Excessive gas. Nausea of pregnancy without vomiting, and worse when walking.

Rectum: Painful hemorrhoids with stitching pains and profuse bleeding. Feels better when sitting on a hard seat. Also relieved by cold. Hemorrhoids often protrude from rectum.

Female: Breasts sore before menses. Flow is premature or weak, acrid and itching. Constant sensation of bearing down.

Soreness in genitals before, during and after menses.

Lungs: Bronchitis; whole chest is very sensitive. Wheezing. Asthma or cough attacks between 2:00 a.m. and 4:00 a.m. Sharp stitching chest pains. Can't lie down; often buries face in pillow while resting on knees instead. Full of phlegm in asthma (unlike more dry Arsenicum Album wheezing).

Back: Small of back feels weak. Back and legs give out. Pains in knees.

Uses

1. Abdominal Pain
2. Asthma
3. Hemorrhoids
4. Indigestion

5. Menstrual Problems
6. Nausea and Vomiting
7. Respiratory Infections
    b. Coughs and Colds

KALI MURIATICUM
(Potassium Chloride) (Kali Mur)

Characteristics

Useful in patients with white bodily discharges. Corresponds generally to the second stage of inflammation when fluid is accumulating and pus is beginning to form. Kali Mur is useful in ear problems; ears feel full, decrease in hearing due to swelling. Often there are snapping, cracking sounds on blowing the nose or swallowing.

Clinical Picture

Ears:	Deafness or earache from congestion and swelling of middle ear or eustachian tubes.
Nose:	White, thick discharge.
Tongue:	Gray-white, coated.
Throat:	Whitish-gray spots on enlarged tonsils; pain on swallowing.
Female:	Non-irritating, milky-white mucus.

Uses

1. Abscesses and
     Inflammation
2. Bleeding
3. Chicken Pox
4. Ear Problems
5. Fever
6. Hayfever
7. Injuries
     d. Burns
8. Mumps
9. Respiratory Infections
     b. Coughs and Colds
     d. Sore Throats
10. Styes
11. Vaginitis

KREOSOTUM
(Beechwood Kreosote)

Characteristics
Known for marked irritation of mucous membranes severe enough to cause ulceration and tissue decay with yellow-white, offensive discharges. Irritated tissues bleed easily from least touch.

Modalities
Worse:	Touch. Cold. At rest or lying.
Better:	Warmth. Sitting (vaginal discharge).

Clinical picture
Mouth:	Ulcerated gums with putrid odor, easily bleed when membrane irritated by contact.
Urinary:	Frequent urging night and day to pass large amounts of pale urine. Often bland discharge from genitalia just before urination. Urine burns genitalia on passing. Incontinence with cough, wets bed. Incontinence is worse lying down.
Female:	Lumpy, gushing, offensive, corrosive, burning, yellow-white discharge sometimes with odor of fresh green corn. Prickling pains between labia. Pain worse with urination. Intercourse painful, may result in bloody discharge. Dragging-down sensation in back with outward pressure in genitalia (like Sepia). Unlike Sepia, however, there is relief from motion.

Uses

1. Urinary Problems
2. Vaginitis

LACHESIS
(Venom of the Bushmaster Snake of South America)

Characteristics
Many symptoms tend to be left-sided. Cannot bear tight clothing. Symptoms worse on awakening. Symptoms relieved with onset of menstrual flow.

Modalities
Worse: Pressure; constriction; touch. After sleep. Heat; hot weather.

Better: Release of pressure. Eating fruit. Cold. Discharges.

Clinical Picture
Mental: Overly talkative; impatient; sad; jealous.

Head: Hammering; sun headaches; weight or pressure on vertex. Headache will awaken the person.

Face: Intense pain in face (maxillary sinus) which comes on when purulent drainage from sinus has stopped. Tends to affect left sinus more than right.

Throat: As if lump in throat; worse on left; hot drinks aggravate (hot drinks help with Hepar Sulph, Lycopodium and Arsenicum Album). Cold drinks alleviate the pain. Worse swallowing liquids. Pain goes to ear on swallowing.

Rectum: Diarrhea before menses with pain. Violet-colored hemorrhoids, very sensitive to contact; pain relieved by bleeding.

Female: Scant, dark, lumpy, offensive menstrual flow. Pains in hips with bearing-down pain in region of left ovary. Pain relieved with onset of menstrual flow. Cannot bear tight clothing around abdomen. Throbbing headaches; dizziness; cramps in chest; aching in stomach before menses. Abdominal spasms during flow.

Lungs: Short, dry cough; averse to anything tight around the neck or chest. Sensation of suffocation whenever lying down. Feels relief after coughing up watery phlegm. Attacks often awaken the patient in the morning or can occur on going to bed.

Uses

1. Asthma
2. Headache
3. Hemorrhoids
4. Menstrual Problems

5. Respiratory Infections
    b. Coughs and Colds
    c. Sinus Infections
    d. Sore Throat

LEDUM PALUSTRE
(Marsh Tea) (Ledum)

Characteristics

Although it has other uses, Ledum is commonly used for stabs and puncture wounds from sharp, pointed instruments, from animal bites and from certain insect bites. It is for the particular pain associated with such wounds, especially if wounded parts are cold, yet pain is relieved by cold application.

It follows Arnica well for cases of severe local bruising and black eyes which do not respond fully to Arnica (compare with Hypericum).

Uses

1. Eye Disorders
2. Injuries
   a. Bites, Stings and Puncture Wounds
   b. Bruises

LYCOPODIUM CLAVATUM
(Club Moss) (Lycopodium)

Characteristics
Digestive disorders; gradual onset of ailments; right-sided symptoms that characteristically shift to the left side of the body. Many symptoms tend to be worse on the right side.

Modalities
Worse: Heat; 4:00 p.m. to 8:00 p.m.
Better: Gentle motion. Open air.

Clinical Picture
Mental: Fears of breaking down under stress; fears of failure; fears of being alone, but does not want anyone near; sensitive to noise, odors; annoyed by trifles.

Head: Headaches, usually right-sided and accompanied by stomach complaints; alternate with thick, yellow nasal discharge.

Nose: Obstruction.

Throat: Inflammation; worse on right side. Better with hot drinks or hot food.

Stomach: Easily feels full. Sense of distress in stomach immediately after eating. Complaints better with hot food and drink. Much belching.

Abdomen: Swollen; better by passing gas. Can't bear pressure of clothing.

Rectum: Constipation frequent; ineffectual urging. When stool has passed there is often sensation as if a large amount still remains.

Urinary: Frequent urination at night; infrequent and small amount during day. Urine of dark

color, may leave red sediment in diaper or
bedsheet. When larger amounts passed,
may be pale and clear with or without
sediment. Foamy urine. May have blood.
Pain in back before urination, causing
crying out. Pain relieved by urination.
Lycopodium is a common remedy for
problems associated with kidney stones or
gravel.

Uses

1. Abdominal Pain
2. Headache
3. Indigestion

4. Respiratory Infections
    d. Sore Throat
5. Urinary Problems

MAGNESIA PHOSPHORICA
(Magnesium Phosphate) (Magnesia Phos)

Characteristics
To relieve sudden spasmodic pains, especially menstrual cramps and abdominal pain. Indicated in muscle cramps and constrictive pains. Compare with Colocynthis for abdominal pains.

Modalities
Worse: Cold. Light. Touch. Night.
Better: Bending over. External warmth. Pressure.

Clinical Picture
Head: Pains shooting, shifting, spasmodic; better by external warmth.
Face: Spasmodic pain.
Tongue: Clean.
Teeth: Toothache, shooting pains relieved by warmth.
Abdomen: Pain with gas, forcing patient to double over to get relief. Better with rubbing, warmth, belching, drawing legs up.
Back: Aching, boring, darting pains anywhere.

Uses

1. Abdominal Pain
2. Headache
3. Hiccough
4. Menstrual Problems
5. Toothache

MANGANUM
(Manganese)

Characteristics
Catches cold easily. The slightest cold seems to find its way into the chest. Bones may be sensitive to touch. Pains in various parts of the body, especially the voicebox, often refer pain to the ears.

Modalities
Worse:	Humidity; cold; before a storm.
Better:	Lying down (cough).

Clinical picture
Nose:	Blowing nose is painful.
Mouth:	Chronic hoarseness. Larynx dry, rough, constricted. Hoarseness is worse in the morning and better after hawking up lumps of mucus. Hoarseness is peculiarly made better by smoking.
Lungs:	Cough triggered by such things as sustained talking, loud reading, or, peculiarly, by scratching the ear canal.

Uses

1. Hoarseness
2. Respiratory Infections
      b. Coughs and Colds

MERCURIUS SOLUBILIS
(Quicksilver) (Merc Sol)

Characteristics

Indicated when trouble has already developed. Adapted for people who are very sensitive to heat or cold weather changes. Swollen glands; profuse sweat which does not relieve; bodily excretions often foul, including pus, sweat, breath, stools. Thin, green-yellow discharges, often profuse and excoriating.

Modalities

Worse: Night; perspiration; wet, damp weather; lying on right side; warmth of bed.

Better: With rest.

Clinical Picture

Nose: Sneezing; nostrils raw, reddened by nasal discharge; thin initially, then thick, yellow-green.

Mouth: Metallic taste; increased saliva; inflamed gums; sharp, pulsating toothache, radiating to ears. Yellow-coated tongue with teeth marks on side; foul breath.

Throat: Sore; inflamed.

Stomach: Intense thirst for cold drinks.

Stool: Green; bloody; slimy; painful; worse at night. Pain unrelieved by passing stool.

Urinary: Sudden urge to urinate. Green pus-filled discharge (suspicious for gonorrhea), especially at night with much burning and swelling of urethral opening. Burning between urination also. May have involuntary urination in bed. Urine can be

	copious or can come out drop by drop. May have blood in urine.
Female:	Profuse discharge always worse at night; greenish or thick; white; corrosive; itching; with relief of itching from washing with cold water. Swelling redness very sensitive to touch. Weakens the person, especially in discharges before puberty.
Lungs:	Cough with yellow-green sputum.
Fever:	Perspiration gives no relief.
Skin:	Constantly moist; glands swollen. Used after Belladonna when pus has formed. Swollen glands. Thin, green pus. Slow formation of pus; pain worse at night. For tonsillar abscess with putrid breath odor.

Uses: Do NOT use with Silica.

1. Abscesses and
      Inflammation
2. Chicken Pox
3. Diarrhea
4. Ear Problems
5. Respiratory Infections
      b. Coughs and Colds
      d. Sore Throats

6. Toothache
7. Urinary Problems
8. Vaginitis

NATRUM MURIATICUM
(Sodium Chloride, Table Salt) (Natrum Mur)

Characteristics

Cold, sensitive people who catch cold easily. More suited to thin people, especially thinness around the neck. Emaciation and dehydration with acute ailments. Tend to be exhausted with throbbing sensations and heart palpitations from any exertion of mind or body. Consolation aggravates symptoms and will often make the person angry. Mucus secretions are normal in character but greatly increased in amount. Despite the copious secretions, there is a marked sense of dryness of mucus membranes. Ailments can come on after emotional upsets, especially disappointments. Also, symptoms arise from loss of bodily fluids (like China).

Modalities

Worse:	Consolation; mid-morning; warmth (despite cold sensitivity); intellectual work.
Better:	Open air.

Clinical Picture

Mind:	Irritability at trifles, especially when consoled. Sadness, especially before menses.
Head:	Headache worse using the mind. Throbbing headache often starts in mid-morning like small hammers. Headache often accompanied by dry sensation of tongue, feeling like it sticks to roof of mouth. Worse from light and noise. Accompanied by nausea and vomiting and intermittent pulse. Can have stitching pains about eyes; worse moving eyes (like Bryonia). Premenstrual headache that persists after menses.

Eyes:	Smart, burning, with sensation of sand under lids. Spasms, sometimes unable to open eyes. Inflammation with eyes stuck together in the morning. Burning tears.
Nose:	Copious discharge of normal-appearing secretions alternating with dryness. Fits of sneezing. Wings of nose sore, sensitive. Loss of sense of smell and taste.
Mouth:	Constant heat and dryness temporarily relieved by thirst. Mapped tongue with sunken red patches (insular patches).
Stomach:	Great thirst. Desire for salty foods (though may also have an aversion for salt). Averse to eating bread. Heartburn after eating, especially during pregnancy, with acidic risings from stomach. Aching, cramping nausea in the morning. Vomiting of frothy, watery phlegm with morning sickness. Can have sinking sensation with feeling of hard object in stomach.
Rectum:	Diarrhea, when present, can be like water, often with mucus, and will often alternate with constipation that has frequent urging, but scant, hard and broken evacuations.
Urinary:	Frequent urging, day and night, often every hour, with large amounts of urine passed. Cutting pain after urination. Can have discharge of mucus after urination. Smarting of genitalia. Abdomen may contract in spasm after urination.
Female:	Menses often late, scanty. Vaginal dryness. Sore breasts before menses. Vaginal discharge, if present, may be thick and transparent or whitish. Discharge is copious and may itch or irritate. If burning,

greenish discharge occurs, this may indicate gonorrhea and a physician should be consulted. Pimples may occur on genitalia.

Chest: Fluttering palpitations before menses.

Lungs: Cough triggered by mucus from post-nasal drainage. Can also cough from tickling in throat or in pit of stomach (latter often results in bursting headache and sometimes spurts of involuntary urination with cough). Hoarseness from cough.

Back: Backache that is better by lying flat on back or better by pressing firmly against back in sitting position.

Fever: Chill usually starts mid-morning, beginning in small of back and feet. Thirst increases with heat. Aching pains all over. Heat rash. Violent fever. Throbbing headache with fever. Copious sweat relieves headache and other symptoms.

Uses

1. Diarrhea
2. Headache
3. Indigestion
4. Menstrual Problems
5. Nausea and Vomiting
6. Respiratory Infections
        b. Coughs and Colds
7. Urinary Problems
8. Vaginitis

NATRUM PHOSPHORICUM
(Sodium Phosphate) (Natrum Phos)

Characteristics

People who need Natrum Phos often suffer from stomach troubles and abnormal bowel habits; diarrhea (often with greenish tinge and sour-smelling) or constipation. Gas and bloating in abdomen which cannot be relieved by passing gas. Sour risings from stomach to throat. Discharges from various parts of body are in general a golden-yellow color.

Clinical Picture

Mouth: Golden-yellow coating on tongue, throat and roof of mouth.

Stomach: Abdominal pain, especially in children with signs of acidity. Gas, unable to release. Worse after eating.

Uses

1. Abdominal Pain
2. Indigestion

NATRUM SULPHURICUM
(Sodium Sulphate) (Natrum Sulph)

Characteristics
Best suited for asthma, abdominal troubles and especially emotional or mental difficulties arising after a head injury. Useful in problems associated with rainy weather and dampness; patient feels every change from dry to wet weather. May remove excess water and fluid retention from body.

Modalities
Worse: Damp weather; damp basements. Lying on the left side.

Better: Dry weather and environments. Pressure. Change of position.

Clinical Picture
Tongue: May have brownish, thick coating.

Abdomen: Great deal of belching and/or passing of gas. Colic. Rumbling of wind in bowels. Abdominal pain, worse from tight clothing and from laying on left side.

Stool: Gushing, watery diarrhea accompanied with much gas.

Urinary: Burning on urination during and after urinating. Frequent urging with scanty urination. On retaining urine, can have pain in small of back. Dark urine can have yellow or brick-dust type sediment.

Lungs: Asthma brought on by, or made worse by, dampness (compare with Dulcamara). May worsen and wake the patient at 4:00 a.m. or 5:00 a.m. Rattling in chest with thick expectoration.

Limbs: Swelling from fluid retention in ankles, feet
             or hands. "Rheumatism" with aching or
             stiffness of joints made worse by dampness.

Uses

1. Abdominal Pain
2. Asthma
3. Diarrhea
4. Urinary Problems

NUX VOMICA
(Poison Nut)

Characteristics
Remedy for overindulgence. Adapted especially to thin, irritable, energetic persons who attend with great detail to tasks; quarrelsome; nervous; intelligent; hypochondriacal; oversensitive to noise, music, light; craves stimulants.

Modalities
Worse:	Overeating; coffee; tobacco; mental over-exertion; sensory stimulation (sight, sound, touch).
Better:	Wet weather; lying down; uninterrupted nap.

Clinical Picture
Head:	Aching, worse in sunshine; accompanied by irritable feeling. Cold air aggravates. Good for hangovers with headache.
Nose:	Dry, stuffy; sneezes in sun or immediately upon waking.
Tongue:	First half clean; posterior fur; white edges.
Throat:	Dry, scraped; worse in morning and in late evening and after overeating.
Stomach:	Nausea, worse in morning and after eating; sensitive to pressure.
Abdomen:	Pain a few hours after eating; bruised soreness; feels like stones rubbed together inside.
Rectal:	Urging frequent but not able to have stool. Constipation occurs reflexively, such as a reaction to labor pains.
Urinary:	Pain before urination, sometimes aborts urge to urinate. Pain can be at base of

bladder with painful urination drop by drop. May have burning pain before, during and after urination. Urge to urinate also creates urge for passing stool. Can also have pattern of frequent passage of pale, watery urine with thick mucus passing during and after urination. Urine can be cloudy with dirty yellow or brick-dust sediment. Can have pain in kidney with inability to lie on affected side.

Female: Dark menses accompanied by retching, abdominal cramps and fainting, especially if in warm room. Breasts tender before menses.

Lungs: Asthma, worse with full stomach, overeating.

Uses

1. Abdominal Pain
2. Asthma
3. Diarrhea
4. Hayfever
5. Headache
6. Hemorrhoids
7. Indigestion

8. Menstrual Problems
9. Nausea and Vomiting
10. Respiratory Infections
    b. Coughs and Colds
    d. Sore Throats
11. Travel Sickness
12. Urinary Problems

PHOSPHORUS

Characteristics

Useful in acute illness for respiratory infections, digestive disorders and skin problems. Tendency to heavy bleeding. Also for nervous disorders especially for artistic temperament and for those easily affected by external stimuli like thunderstorms, weather changes, odors, loud noises. Often needed by thin, narrow-chested people.

Modalities

Worse: Physical or mental exertion; night; warm food or drink; weather changes; during thunderstorms; getting wet in hot weather; lying on left side.

Better: Lying on right side; cold; open air; sleep.

Clinical Picture

Mental: Spacey; overly sensitive; fearful.

Eyes: Flashes; colors; light seen before vision.

Nose: Nose bleeds; overly sensitive to bad odors.

Mouth: Very thirsty for cold water.

Stomach: Post-operative vomiting after anesthesia; hungry soon after eating; hunger with fever; vomits cold water after it gets warm in stomach.

Abdomen: Painless, copious diarrhea causing great weakness; hemorrhoids bleed profusely.

Lungs: Laryngitis; cannot talk because of pain in larynx; cough made worse by tickling feeling, cold air, talking, reading; cough or bronchitis comes on after weather changes; cough worse lying on left side.

Sleep: Dreams of fire; short naps with frequent waking.

| Fever: | Fever with increased appetite. |
| Skin: | Wounds bleed easily; black and blue spots. |

Uses

1. Bleeding
2. Diarrhea
3. Fever
4. Hemorrhoids
5. Hoarseness
6. Indigestion

7. Injuries
   c. Bites, Stings and
    Puncture Wounds
8. Nausea and Vomiting
9. Respiratory Infections
   b. Colds and Coughs

PHYTOLACCA
(Poke Root)

Characteristics
Pre-eminently a glandular remedy. Swollen glands with heat and inflammation. Soreness and aching, usually of throat or breasts.

Modalities
Worse:	Swallowing; right side; hot drinks; cold, damp nights.
Better:	Cold drinks; dry weather; warmth; rest.

Clinical Picture
Mental:	Preoccupied with pain.
Eyes:	Hot tears.
Throat:	Dark bluish-red appearance. Tonsils swollen. Shooting pains into ears upon swallowing. Cannot swallow anything hot. Mumps. Stiff neck.
Breasts:	Premenstrual breast pain that forms hard lumps or for plugged ducts during breastfeeding when pain radiates to armpit.

Uses

1. Menstrual Problems
2. Respiratory Infections
    d. Sore Throats

PODOPHYLLUM
(May Apple)

Characteristics

Affects chiefly the duodenum of the small intestines and the rectum. Mainly used in diarrhea and vomiting, especially of infants.

Modalities

Worse: Early morning; eating; hot weather; teething; too much acidic fruit.

Better: Massaging abdomen; lying on abdomen.

Clinical Picture

Stomach: Gagging, vomiting and/or empty retching; weak, empty, sinking or sick feeling in abdomen. Thirst for large quantities of cold water (Bryonia).

Rectum: Gurgling through bowels, then profuse, putrid stools gush out painlessly. Early morning diarrhea (may drive out of bed) during teething with hot glowing cheeks. Profuse watery stool with jelly-like mucus.

Uses

1. Abdominal Pain
2. Diarrhea

PULSATILLA NIGRICANS
(Pulsatilla) (Wood Flower)

Characteristics

Remedy often indicated in those with mild, gentle, timid, yielding dispositions, who are easily moved to laughter and tears. The Pulsatilla person wants to be held and loved; moods changeable and fickle. Patient is chilly, but desires strolling in open air. Symptoms are erratic, change frequently. Most distinctive pains of Pulsatilla patient are wandering pains and pains that grow gradually in intensity. Fever without thirst, despite dry mouth. Bland, yellow discharges.

Modalities

Worse: Evening before midnight; warmth (room, applications or coverings); after eating fat, rich food.

Better: Open air; cold applications; consolation relieves symptoms.

Clinical Picture

Eyes: Bland pus, worse at night with lids stuck together on waking. Highly inflamed styes. Frequently needed for conjunctivitis of infants.

Ears: Sensation as if something were being forced outward; difficulty hearing, as if ears were stuffed. Earache better from cool applications.

Nose: Yellow, usually non-irritating mucus abundant in morning; stoppage in evening.

Mouth: Dry mouth without thirst.

Tongue: Yellow or white, covered with tenacious mucus.

Stomach: Averse to fat, warm food and drink. Vomits clear yellow liquid in morning, especially with morning sickness of pregnancy.

Urinary: Frequent or constant ineffectual desire to urinate associated with paroxysmal pains. Urine may escape if unable to get to bathroom shortly after urge occurs. Worse from exposure to cold or dampness. Worse lying on back. Pain in bladder if urge is postponed. Burning in neck (outlet above urethra) of bladder during urination. Urine burning, cloudy, dark, ammonia smelling, bloody, mucus or purulent (pus).

Female: Delayed start of flow, especially at onset of puberty. Changeable flow, starting and stopping, ranging from dark clots to colorless water. Breasts sore. Cramping pains, can hardly tolerate them. Feels smothered in a closed room. Can help with afterpains of pregnancy also. Vaginal discharge usually thick, like cream (especially in children), and bland, but discharge may also change and be watery and corrosive with cutting pains and external swelling.

Lungs: Dry cough evening and night, especially before 10:00 p.m., just on going to bed. Yellow, green, bland mucus, easy to cough up.

Uses

1. Asthma
2. Chicken Pox
3. Ear Problems
4. Fever
5. Headache
6. Hemmorhoids
7. Indigestion
8. Measles
9. Menstrual Problems
10. Mumps
11. Nausea and Vomiting
12. Respiratory Infections
    b. Coughs and Colds
13. Styes
14. Toothache
15. Urinary Problems
16. Vaginitis

PYROGENIUM
(Pyrogen)

Characteristics

Useful when septic states (systemic spread of bacterial infection) threaten. Great aching, cannot lie for more than a few minutes in any one position.

Modalities

Worse: Lying still.
Better: Better temporarily by change in position.

Clinical Picture

Fever: May commence with pains in the limbs. Perspiration has odor of dead animal. Shivering common at times, accompanied by desire to move.

Uses

1. Abscesses and Inflammation
2. Fevers
3. Toothache

RHODODENDRON
(Dwarf Rosebag) (Snow-Rose)

Characteristics
Used for pains, especially when occur before a storm.

Modalities:
Worse: Worse before a storm; by cold humid weather. At rest.

Better: After a storm; by dry heat. Motion. Wrapping up.

Clinical Picture
Teeth: Tearing, jerking pains; better with food and warmth; worse before storms. Pain worse in bed.

Limbs: Rheumatic pains worse before a storm, by humid cold and at rest.

Uses

1. Toothache

RHUS TOXICODENDRON
(Poison Oak) (Rhus Toxicodendron)

Characteristics
Patient is extremely restless; frequent change of position which temporarily improves pains and anxiety; mainly affects joints and muscles. Irritability mentally.

Modalities
Worse: Sleep; cold, wet weather; night; at rest.
Better: Brief relief with change of position; warm, dry weather; warm applications; continued movement.

Clinical Picture
Face: Jaw cracks; glands swollen and painful; mumps with restlessness.
Stomach: Nausea with dizziness from travelling.
Stool: Blood and/or mucus with diarrhea.
Lungs: Hoarseness from overusing voice; dry, teasing cough—more after midnight.
Limbs: Tearing pains in ligaments, tendons and muscles; swelling in joints; pains relieved by gentle motion; better with warm applications.
Skin: Itching, with small fluid-filled bubbles (vesicles) grouped together in clumps with surrounding inflammation. Red, swollen eruptions like Chicken Pox or Poison Ivy. Itching better with warm applications.

Uses

1. Chicken Pox
2. Diarrhea
3. Hoarseness
4. Injuries
    e. Sprains and Strains
5. Mumps
6. Poison Ivy or Oak
7. Respiratory Infections
    b. Coughs and Colds
8. Skin Diseases
9. Travel Sickness

RUMEX CRISPUS
(Yellow Dock)

Characteristics
Affects respiratory membranes. Catches cold easily. Covers nose and mouth to protect. Always looking for warmth.

Modalities
Worse:　　　Cold. Breathing cold air. Undressing. Evening.
Better:　　　Warmth.

Clinical Picture
Rectum:　　　At the end of, or after, a cold brings painless, uncontrollable diarrhea with sudden profuse, foul stool. Diarrhea usually occurs from 5 a.m. to 10 a.m.

Lungs:　　　Dry, tiring, continuous cough triggered by irritation under the breastbone (sternum). Burning in voicebox or windpipe. Hoarseness worse in evening. Can hawk up tenacious mucus.

Skin:　　　Itching on undressing or exposure to cold, but without rash. Itching is better with warmth.

Uses

1. Diarrhea
2. Respiratory Infections
    b. Coughs and Colds

RUTA GRAVEOLENS
(Rue-Bitterwort) (Ruta)

Characteristics

Used in sprains, after Arnica, when site of injury seems to be where tendons join the bone. Hard deposits may be formed at site of injury near bone.

Modalities

Worse: Cold, wet weather; lying down; every motion of affected part (compare with Rhus Toxicodendron).

Clinical Picture

Head: Headache after eye strain; eyes are red, hot, tired, especially after prolonged close work such as sewing or reading small print.

Limbs: Pain feels closer to the bone, such as the shin or wrist, and can be associated with hard swelling where the tendon is attached to the bone. Pain is aching in character and is made worse by every movement of the injured part. Alleviates pain and tenderness when bruise occurs close to bone.

Uses

1. Headache
2. Injuries
    c. Bruises
    e. Sprains and Strains

SEPIA
(Inky Juice of the Cuttlefish)

Characteristics

Exhausted; dragging-downward sensations; generally better in the afternoon; worse in the morning and in the evening. Disturbed circulation with frequent flushes. Easily out of balance because of sensitivity, delicateness of condition. Often pale, flabby persons with fair, but flushed skin. Takes cold easily at change of weather as part of sensitivities. Sensitive to external influences such as touch, jarring. Vigorous exercise, however, sometimes improves some symptoms. Ailments from sexual excess. Particularly prone to problems of sexual organs. Stomach has an empty, all-gone sensation in the late morning like Sulphur, but without the accompanying urgent hunger of Sulphur.

Modalities

Worse: Morning; evening; sensory stimuli such as touch, light, noise; approach of violent weather.

Better: Afternoon. Exercise.

Clinical Picture

Head: Sharp pain in lower part of brain extending upward, which brings on vomiting. Another pattern is that of throbbing over eye (usually left) accompanied by flashes of heat in head, especially with motion. Worse light, noise.

Eyes: Discharge of pus or dry scabs on lids in morning, relatively comfortable in daytime, and uncomfortable dryness in evening. Inflammation with redness of whites of eyes. Styes common. Better with cold washing and in hot weather. Can be sensitive to light, especially to reflected light off bright objects.

Face: Yellow coloring with headache (pale with Pulsatilla). Can also have pale, flabby appearance.

Mouth: Sour, bitter taste. White tongue.

Stomach: Gone, empty feeling. May crave acids and pickles to relieve taste in mouth. Morning sickness relieved by eating.

Urinary: Aching pressure in bladder with frequent desire to urinate. Can have involuntary urination during first part of sleep. Offensive, cloudy urine with uric acid sediment.

Female: Morning sickness relieved by eating. Bearing-down pain in abdomen and small of back. Organs feel as if forced out through vulva, though some relief on sitting with legs crossed. Worse if standing or walking. Gripping pain as if suddenly seized by a hand. This pain or burning pain may shoot upward. Menses is usually late and scant. Yellow-green, offensive, often excoriating discharge.

Lungs: Dryness of voicebox and windpipe, tickling in either of which can trigger cough. Dryness sufficient to cause hoarseness. Cough brings up yellow-green, putrid or salty mucus, usually in morning and evening with some relief in afternoon and at night. If cough occurs at night, can be with suffocation and retching, which weakens one. Can be worse lying on left side.

Limbs: Hands hot, feet cold, or vice versa.

Skin: Poison Ivy eruption is better in a warm
             room but aggravated by warmth of the bed.

Uses

1. Headache
2. Menstrual Problems
3. Nausea and Vomiting
4. Poison Ivy

5. Respiratory Infections
    b. Coughs and Colds
6. Urinary Problems
7. Vaginitis

SILICEA
(Silicon dioxide) (Pure Flint)

Characteristics

Use cautiously. Ripens abscesses; promotes drainage of pus, once pus appears and no new material is found in the boil or abscess. If tenderness is present with the abscess, consider Hepar Sulph or other remedies first.

Useful in earache or sinus infections to complete drainage and restore hearing or help ruptured eardrum heal. Eardrum can have characteristic appearance of redness around the rim.

Uses

1. Abscesses and Inflammation
2. Ear Problems
3. Respiratory Infections
        c. Sinus Infections
4. Styes

SPONGIA TOSTA
(Roasted Sponge) (Spongia)

Characteristics

Used in symptoms of respiratory organs; cough, croup; anxiety and difficulty breathing. Exhaustion of body after slight exertion.

Modalities

Worse: Ascending; wind; cold; before midnight.
Better: Descending; head low.

Clinical Picture

Lungs: Dryness of air passages; burning of larynx (voicebox), which is sensitive to touch; feels as if plug is stuck there. Croup worse during inspiration and before midnight. Cough better after eating or drinking, especially warm drinks. Wheezing, worse in cold air with increased phlegm.

Uses

1. Respiratory Infections
     a. Croup
     b. Coughs and Colds

STICTA PULMONARIA
(Lungwort) (Sticta)

Characteristics
Used for respiratory symptoms: coughs with head colds, sneezing; stiffness; joint pains often present. Weariness.

Modalities
Worse: Sudden change of temperature; evening; inspiration.

Clinical picture
Nose: Pressure or fullness at root of nose. Dry, but constant inclination to blow nose. Incessant sneezing.

Throat: Dryness, especially back roof of mouth (soft palate). Postnasal drip makes throat raw. Painful to swallow. Swollen glands and external soreness, especially left side.

Lungs: Cough dry, hacking during night, can be croupy. Worse inspiration. Prevents sleep. Tickling in larynx or windpipe. Cough can be spasmodic, feels like it can't be stopped once it starts.

Uses

1. Respiratory Infections
     b. Coughs and Colds

SULPHUR

Characteristics

Key symptoms which may correspond with any problem requiring Sulphur include: flushes of heat, with heat on top of the head, cold feet (though may feel burning to patient), and sinking feeling in stomach. Openings to the body may be distinctly red, including margins of lids, lips, ears, anus. Perspiration tends to be absent or foul smelling. Generally not indicated as a first remedy. Patient is often dirty, disorganized or messy.

Modalities

Worse:　Heat; bathing; warmth of bed; stooping.
Better:　Open air; uncovering.

Clinical Picture

Eye:　Red margins; foreign body sensation (like sand or splinter). Worse near heat.

Ear:　Itchy. Ear lobes may be red with face pale. May have roaring in ears.

Nose:　Stuffed indoors. Open outdoors. May have red scabbiness in side wings of nose. Bleeds easily.

Throat:　Hoarseness with low voice or absence of voice, especially in morning. Sore throat better with warm drinks.

Lungs:　Seldom indicated in initial stage of cold but may resolve cases having difficulty clearing up lingering mucus involvement. Cough worse lying down.

Stomach:　Sour vomiting mixed with undigested food. Empty feeling at 11:00 a.m. with hunger. May not tolerate milk. Morning sickness of pregnancy without vomiting, but with faint, sick spells mid to late morning and taste like vomitus in mouth. Especially averse to meat at that time.

Abdomen: Tightness after small quantities of food.

Stool: Diarrhea drives from bed (in early morning). Constipation alternates with diarrhea. Hemorrhoids itch, burn and bleed.

Female: Weak, heavy feeling with bearing-down pains above pubic bone in lower abdomen. Pains may run from groin to back. Can have abdominal spasms, headache accompanying. Flashes of heat often accompany uterine symptoms, as does an aversion to washing the area. Inflammation of genitals with pimple-like eruption. Corrosive, offensive, yellowish discharge with pain preceding. Morning sickness of pregnancy without vomiting, but with faint, sick spells in the mid to late morning and a taste like vomitus in the mouth. Especially averse to meat during the morning sickness.

Limbs: Jerking of limbs on falling asleep. Pain worse in bed at night.

Fever: Desires to be uncovered. Child may thrust limbs out of covers. Dry, hot skin with constant fever though may have slight fall in temperature toward morning and worsen each evening.

Skin: Acrid, burning pus.

Uses

1. Abscesses and
   Inflammation
2. Diarrhea
3. Hoarseness
4. Menstrual Problems
5. Nausea and Vomiting

6. Respiratory Infections
   b. Coughs and Colds
   c. Sinus Infections
   d. Sore Throats
7. Vaginitis

SYMPHYTUM
(Comfrey Root)

Generalities

Mainly used for musculoskeletal problems where there is injury with disruption of the outer layer of bone (periosteum) causing pricking, sticking pains and slow healing (including inability of ends of fractured bones to knit together). Such disruption can occur where there is a fracture, or where the tendon attachment is partially or completely detached from the bone.

Clinical picture

Eyes: Blunt trauma to the eye without injury to the surrounding area.

Uses

1. Injuries

TABACUM
(Tobacco)

Characteristics
Travel Sickness with vertigo and vomiting. Icy cold sweats. Death-like paleness of face and sensation of weakness. Hiccoughs and coughs occur together leading to a sense of suffocation.

Modalities
Worse: Extremes of temperature, both hot and cold. Rising up; looking upwards.

Better: Uncovering. Fresh air. Uncovering the abdomen.

Clinical Picture
Stomach: Persistent nausea, vomiting and vertigo. Seasickness with vomiting; worse from the least bodily motion; better on deck in fresh, cold air. Nausea worse from the smell of tobacco smoke. Increased saliva with the nausea, especially in pregnancy. Sinking feeling in pit of stomach. Child wants abdomen uncovered, which relieves nausea and vomiting.

Lungs: Dry cough with hiccoughs during or after the cough. May vomit with the cough. Intense hiccoughs, as if one would suffocate. Cannot take a deep breath.

Uses
1. Nausea and Vomiting
2. Respiratory Infections
    b. Coughs and Colds

3. Travel Sickness

URTICA URENS
(Dwarf Stinging Nettle)

Characteristics
Common uses are skin and urinary complaints in acute prescribing.

Modalities
Worse: Cold applications (opposite of Apis); touch. Skin symptoms often worse after sleep.

Clinical Picture
Urinary: Acrid urine, causing itching. Itching, burning genitalia. Useful for attacks of urinary colic from uric-acid stones, especially if accompanied by fever.

Skin: Prickly heat rash with sweatiness and small vesicles (fluid-filled, pimple-like eruptions). Prickly burning with swelling and severe itching, worse cold applications and bathing or washing. Hives are smaller than Apis. Apis is also better with cold, not worse.

Uses

1. Skin Diseases
2. Urinary Problems

VERATRUM ALBUM
(White Hellebore)

Characteristics
Copious discharges. Coldness, inside and externally. Pain compels to move, but no relief from motion. Exhaustion and faintness.

Modalities
Worse: Cold; cold, wet weather.
Better: Heat.

Clinical Picture
Head: Worse rising; better external pressure and bending head backwards. Scalp sensitive; may feel hot and cold at same time.

Nose: Dryness; sensation of painful ulceration. Violent, frequent sneeze. May smell burnt odor.

Mouth: Painful ulcers; salivation; dryness.

Face: May have one side pale, and the other flushed (Chamomilla, Pulsatilla).

Throat: Dry, constricting pain on swallowing.

Stomach: Bitter vomiting after meal. Hunger with nausea. Vomiting and stool at same time.

Bowel: Onset of diarrhea may follow drinking cold fluids on hot day or after fright (Gelsemium, Aconite). Green, profuse watery stool, sometimes with flakes resembling spinach. Podophyllum stools in contrast are painless, variable color and more forceful.

Lungs: Dryness of nose, palate, mouth and throat. Tickling deep in trachea or chest excites cough. Cough worse with cold food or

drink. Pain inside inguinal ring with cough.
May vomit with cough. Worse evening and
morning. May have easy expectoration or
dryness.

Limbs: Icy cold. Painful stiffness, worse mornings
or after walking.

Fever: Coldness even when warmly covered. Parts
stay cold during fever. Cold sweat on
forehead.

Uses

1. Diarrhea
2. Respiratory Infections
     b. Coughs and Colds

VERBASCUM
(Mullein Flower)

Characteristics

Generally for earaches. Can be given as eardrops made from tincture prepared with olive oil, or can be given in potency.

Modalities

Worse: Night; cough.
Better: Deep breathing, especially cough.

Clinical Picture

Ear: Pain with face ache.
Face: Squeezing, cramping, paralyzing face ache in malar bones, which are below the eyes and joining the nose. Affects particularly the left side. Feels worse with change of temperature, especially warm to cold. Worse at night and with cough.
Lungs: Deep, hollow, hoarse, barking cough. Does not awaken from cough. Cough is better with deep breathing.

Uses

1. Ear Problems
2. Respiratory Infections
        b. Coughs and Colds

Section 4

Repertory Graphs

INTRODUCTION

This section is written to further assist the prescriber in learning to repertorize the signs and symptoms of an illness and to understand the importance of comparative materia medica. Here the computer-assisted repertorization is displayed in visually pleasing graphs, allowing the prescriber to quickly view which remedies are more common for an ailment and how many remedies share in the same symptom.

Repertorizing a case is the art of selecting key signs and symptoms of an illness and matching them to a remedy. The repertory and the materia medica are the two major references used for this task. The *Materia Medica* (Section 3) contains the signs and symptoms of the remedies as derived from the original provings of the remedy. The *Clinical Repertory* (Section 2) relates the remedies to specific signs and symptoms. A *rubric* is a listing of these signs or symptoms followed by the remedies.

For the past 75 years the *Repertory of the Homeopathic Materia Medica* by James Tyler Kent (1849-1916) was considered the most complete and reliable repertory. Only in the last few years has computer technology entered the world of homeopathy. The powerful personal computers revolutionized homeopathic repertorization and resources, surpassing the monumental works of Kent and others.

The repertory graphs in this book were designed by the MacRepertory© computer program, utilizing Roger van Zandvoort's *Complete Repertory*; this expanded version of Kent's Repertory contains 200,000 new additions along with 45,000 new rubrics.

To the experienced homeopath, this means they will find new insights and uses for remedies in the following pages. For the newcomer to homeopathy, this means this text will introduce you to the most reliable and appropriate uses for homeopathy within the scope and context of this book.

We should further note that we, the authors, found new insights into the remedies thanks to *Reference Works*, a huge computerized compilation of many materia medicas. The materia medica is the source of all repertories, and only recently has computer technology allowed the homeopath to easily verify and correct his repertory knowledge through searches into the original materia medicas.

RUBRICS

Kent realized that some remedies were much more frequently indicated than other remedies for a particular sign or symptom. He used various typestyles in his repertory to represent grades of the remedies. In the following graphs, we have the done the same thing; instead of the bold type of Kent's Repertory, we have bold shading of a box to indicate that the remedy is frequently indicated for that symptom. Kent's remedies that were in plain type are shown in lightly shaded boxes, and his italic listings are shown in medium gray boxes.

The highest importance is a black box with a white dot in the center; however, this highest rating is rare compared with the next level, that of a boldly shaded box.

Kent limited his grading to three levels, but today most repertories are adding a fourth level to reflect great importance of a remedy in a rubric. Kent's bold typeface was his highest level and signified remedies that brought out the symptom in all or a majority of the provers. The italics typeface denoted remedies that brought out the symptom in a few provers.

The ordinary typeface of Kent has two very different interpretations that Kent does not further distinguish. One interpretation is that the remedies only brought out the symptom now and then in provers. The second interpretation is that the remedies have cured the symptom in patients, but did not cause the symptom during the proving. Thus, this lowest grade of Kent may designate remedies that have cured clinical cases even though these symptoms were not produced by that same remedy in the provings.

By examining the grades of the remedy, homeopaths will gain greater precision in their prescribing. For example, if a patient has vomiting relieved by cold water and the prescriber sees Phosphorous listed in a bold box, this is a good sign that Phosphorous will alleviate this condition. Of course, the importance of Phosphorous is dependent upon the relevance of Phosphorous to the entire rubrics of the case.

The signs and symptoms of the illness, called *rubrics*, are listed here in the same order and language of Kent's Repertory. Each rubric is followed by remedies shown with a shaded box that reflects the importance of the remedy within the rubric. The modalities shown in rubrics imply that the condition aggravates the complaint, unless otherwise noted. The most common exception to this rule are rubrics ending with *"amel."* This abbreviation for *ameliorate* is added to the end of a rubric when the complaint is improved or "ameliorated" by the action or condition listed in the rubric.

To illustrate the language of the rubrics, here are two examples. *"Stomach; PAIN; burning; warm drinks"* is a rubric stating that the burning pain in the stomach is aggravated by warm drinks. The next rubric is *"Stomach; PAIN; burning; warm drinks amel."* This rubric states that the burning pain in the stomach is relieved (ameliorated) by warm drinks.

Once the correct rubrics are selected and the grading of the remedies are noted, then the prescriber can recognize the strengths and weaknesses that each remedy has for various signs and symptoms of the case. In general, the ideal repertorization of a case would reveal a single remedy that is found in the fourth degree for all the important rubrics of the case. When this is not possible, studying the unique differences of the remedies in reference to a specific rubric or to the entire case can be considered in the selection of the best remedy for the case.

INTERPRETING THE GRAPHS

The *Remedy* is listed in an abbreviated fashion across the top of the graphs. These abbreviations are universal to homeopathy and allow the reader to refer to the materia medica for complete identification of the remedy.

The *Number of Rubrics* shows how many rubrics are covered by each remedy. This number is listed below the remedy abbreviation in the graph.

The *Number of Different Remedies* is limited by the authors to the remedies found in the *Clinical Repertory* (Section 2) and in the *Materia Medica* (Section 3) of this book. For the most part, remedies were chosen for their wide variety of uses for common ailments. Thus, the layperson can have a home remedy kit that will be useful for many ailments. Remedies that are specific to a particular condition and historically yield results for that ailment are also included in this text.

REPERTORY GRAPHS

The reader should note that some graphs are several pages long. The rubrics are listed as they appear in MacRepertory©, following the format of Kent's Repertory.

In the Abdominal Pain section, as well as others, the term "aching" refers to generalized pain, not to a type of pain that would be described as an "aching" pain. To avoid confusion, the authors have avoided using rubrics where the pain is specifically described as "aching".

There are special sections reflecting the effect of warmth and cold in the Croup, Coughs and Colds section. These graphs depict the rubrics aggravated and ameliorated by temperature extremes.

ABDOMINAL PAIN

Remedy	
Ip.	6
Nat-p.	7
Podo.	10
Acon.	11
Cupr.	13
Nat-s.	13
Mag-p.	13
Cocc.	13
Lyc.	18
Kali-c.	18
Bry.	19
Bell.	20
Ars.	20
Cham.	22
Nux-v.	24
Coloc.	26

Rubrics

1. Mind; SHRIEKING, screaming, shouting; pain, with the
2. Stomach; DISTENTION; eructations; amel.
3. Stomach; PAIN; General; eating; after
4. Stomach; PAIN; General; eating; amel.
5. Stomach; PAIN; burning; warm drinks amel.
6. Stomach; STONE, sensation of
7. Stomach; STONE, sensation of; eating, after
8. Abdomen; DISTENSION
9. Abdomen; DISTENSION; eating; after
10. Abdomen; DISTENSION; flatus, passing; amel.
11. Abdomen; DISTENSION; painful
12. Abdomen; FLATULENCE; obstructed
13. Abdomen; PAIN; aching, dull pain; anger, after
14. Abdomen; PAIN; aching, dull pain; bending; double; amel.
15. Abdomen; PAIN; aching, dull pain; bending; double; must
16. Abdomen; PAIN; aching, dull pain; cold; drinks, after
17. Abdomen; PAIN; aching, dull pain; cold; taking, from and as from
18. Abdomen; PAIN; aching, dull pain; constipation; from
19. Abdomen; PAIN; aching, dull pain; diarrhoea; as if, would come on
20. Abdomen; PAIN; aching, dull pain; diarrhoea; amel.

ABDOMINAL PAIN

Ip. [6]
Nat-p. [7]
Podo. [10]
Acon. [11]
Cupr. [13]
Nat-s. [13]
Mag-p. [13]
Cocc. [13]
Lyc. [18]
Kali-c. [18]
Bry. [19]
Bell. [20]
Ars. [20]
Cham. [22]
Nux-v. [24]
Coloc. [26]

Rubrics

21. Abdomen; PAIN; aching, dull pain; diarrhoea; during
22. Abdomen; PAIN; aching, dull pain; eating; after
23. Abdomen; PAIN; aching, dull pain; flatus; passing; amel.
24. Abdomen; PAIN; aching, dull pain; heat; during
25. Abdomen; PAIN; aching, dull pain; menses; before
26. Abdomen; PAIN; aching, dull pain; menses; beginning of
27. Abdomen; PAIN; aching, dull pain; menses; during
28. Abdomen; PAIN; aching, dull pain; motion; on
29. Abdomen; PAIN; aching, dull pain; pressure; amel.
30. Abdomen; PAIN; aching, dull pain; stool; after; amel.
31. Abdomen; PAIN; aching, dull pain; violent
32. Abdomen; PAIN; aching, dull pain; warmth amel.
33. Abdomen; PAIN; aching, dull pain; warm; drinks amel.
34. Abdomen; PAIN; aching, dull pain; Inguinal region; rising from a seat
35. Abdomen; PAIN; cramping
36. Abdomen; PAIN; cramping; babies, in
37. Abdomen; PAIN; cramping; pressure; amel.
38. Abdomen; PAIN; aching, dull pain; stones, like sharp, rubbing…
39. Abdomen; PAIN; aching, dull pain; as if squeezed between two stones
40. Abdomen; PAIN; sore; jarring; on
41. Abdomen; PAIN; sore; touch; on

ASTHMA

Rubrics	Ars. 20	Lach. 21	Puls. 18	Carb-v. 17	Ip. 18	Nux-v. 17	Kali-c. 15	Ant-t. 15	Nat-s. 13	Arg-n. 13	Kali-bi. 9	Calc-p. 5
1. Mind; FEAR; suffocation, of	X			X								
2. Stomach; GAGGING; coughing, from		X		X		X				X		
3. Stomach; RETCHING; cough, with	X	X	X	X	X	X	X			X		
4. Respiration; ABDOMINAL								X				
5. Respiration; ASTHMATIC; midnight, after	X	X		X								
6. Respiration; ASTHMATIC; anger, after	X						X					
7. Respiration; ASTHMATIC; anxiety, with										X		
8. Respiration; ASTHMATIC; cold; damp weather	X									X		
9. Respiration; ASTHMATIC; eating, after			X									
10. Respiration; ASTHMATIC; emotions, after												
11. Respiration; ASTHMATIC; expectoration amel.						X			X		X	
12. Respiration; DIFFICULT; air; open, in; amel.		X	X				X					
13. Respiration; DIFFICULT; cold; taking, after			X									
14. Respiration; DIFFICULT; eating; after	X	X	X	X	X	X				X		
15. Respiration; DIFFICULT; exertion, after	X	X	X	X			X		X	X		
16. Respiration; DIFFICULT; expectoration; amel.								X				
17. Respiration; DIFFICULT; fanned, wants to be	X	X		X								
18. Respiration; DIFFICULT; lying, while; amel.		X				X					X	
19. Respiration; DIFFICULT; lying, while; impossible	X	X				X						
20. Respiration; DIFFICULT; motion; amel.		X								X		
21. Respiration; DIFFICULT; motion	X								X			
22. Respiration; DIFFICULT; sitting; bent; forward; amel.	X	X										
23. Respiration; DIFFICULT; sitting; upright							X					
24. Respiration; DIFFICULT; sitting; upright; amel.		X						X				
25. Respiration; DIFFICULT; stormy weather	X					X						
26. Respiration; RATTLING	X	X	X	X	X	X		X				X
27. Respiration; RATTLING; expectoration, before; without					X		X					
28. Cough; DRY	X	X	X	X	X	X		X		X		X
29. Cough; LOOSE				X				X				
30. Expectoration; EASY		X	X							X		
31. Expectoration; DIFFICULT	X	X	X		X	X					X	
32. Chest; OPPRESSION	X	X		X		X		X	X	X	X	
33. Generalities; WEATHER; cold, wet; agg.	X	X	X	X		X		X		X		X
34. Generalities; WEATHER; wet; agg.	X	X	X	X		X		X		X		
35. Generalities; WEATHER; wind; ailments from	X	X	X	X		X						

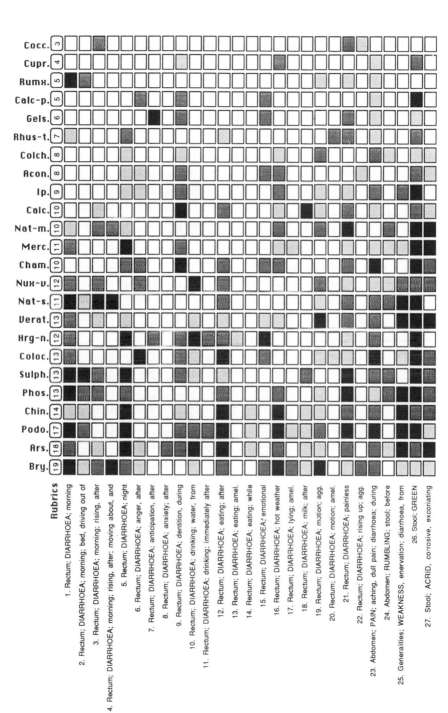

EAR PROBLEMS

Rubrics	Merc.	Puls.	Calc.	Sil.	Hep.	Bell.	Cham.	Acon.	Verb.	Kali-m.
	24	22	23	20	18	13	11	13	6	6
1. Mind; CARRIED, desires to be	▨	▨	▨			▨	■	▨		
2. Mind; CARRIED, desires to be; caressed and, desires to...		▨								
3. Mind; CONSOLATION; amel.		■								
4. Mind; CONSOLATION; kind words agg.	▨		▨		▨	■	▨			
5. Ear; AIR; open, sensitive to, about ears	▨					■	▨	■		
6. Ear; CARIES, threatened			▨	■						
7. Ear; CARIES, threatened; mastoid process			▨	▨						
8. Ear; CATARRH; Eustachian tube	▨	■	▨		▨					▨
9. Ear; CATARRH; middle ear, chronic										▨
10. Ear; DISCHARGES; fetid	■		▨	▨	▨					
11. Ear; DISCHARGES; offensive	▨	▨	▨	■						
12. Ear; DISCHARGES; painful	■									
13. Ear; DISCHARGES; purulent	▨	■	■	■	■	▨	▨	▨		
14. Ear; DISCHARGES; watery	▨		▨							
15. Ear; DISCHARGES; yellow	▨	■	▨	▨						
16. Ear; DISCOLORATION; redness	▨	▨			▨	▨		▨		
17. Ear; GLUE-EAR										▨
18. Ear; INFLAMMATION	■		▨			▨				
19. Ear; INFLAMMATION; media	■	■	■			▨				
20. Ear; MOISTURE; behind ears			▨							
21. Ear; PAIN; General; right	▨	▨					■		▨	
22. Ear; PAIN; General; left		▨							▨	
23. Ear; PAIN; General; air; cold, in					▨			▨		▨
24. Ear; PAIN; General; air; open, in; amel.		▨								
25. Ear; PAIN; General; air; open, in							▨			
26. Ear; PAIN; General; cold; applications; agg.			▨	▨	■					
27. Ear; PAIN; General; cold; applications; amel.	▨									
28. Ear; PAIN; General; cold; taking, from	▨	▨								
29. Ear; PAIN; General; lying; ear, on						▨				
30. Ear; PAIN; General; lying; ear, on; amel.										

EAR PROBLEMS

Rubrics	Merc.	Puls.	Calc.	Sil.	Hep.	Bell.	Cham.	Acon.	Verb.	Kali-m.
	24	22	23	20	18	13	11	13	6	6
31. Ear; PAIN; General; motion, on; amel.							■			
32. Ear; PAIN; General; swallowing, on	■									
33. Ear; PAIN; General; warmth; wrapping up amel., and					■	■				
34. Ear; PERFORATION of tympanum	■		■	■						
35. Ear; STOPPED sensation	■		■	■			■	■	■	
36. Ear; SUPPURATION; middle ear	■	■	■	■						
37. Ear; SWELLING; inside		■		■						
38. Ear; ULCERATION; tympanum	■		■							
39. Hearing; IMPAIRED; catarrh of eustachian tube		■	■		■					■
40. Hearing; IMPAIRED; blowing nose; amel.	■									
41. Hearing; IMPAIRED; leaf or membrane before the ear,...			■		■				■	
42. Generalities; PAIN; appear suddenly		■		■		■		■	■	
43. Generalities; PAIN; appear gradually			■							
44. Generalities; LYING; agg.; side, on; painful	■	■	■	■	■	■		■	■	
45. Generalities; LYING; amel.; side, on; painful		■	■			■	■			

FEVER

Rubrics	Bell.	Ars.	Bry.	Puls.	Acon.	Chin.	Phos.	Gels.	Eup-per.	Apis	Pyrog.	Bapt.	Kali-m.
	25	22	22	20	19	18	16	11	9	9	6	6	2
1. Mind; ANXIETY; fever; during	▨	■	▨	▨	■	░	▨						
2. Mind; CARRIED, desires to be		▨	■										
3. Mind; DELIRIUM	■	■	▨	▨	▨	░	▨	░			░	▨	
4. Mind; DULLNESS; heat; during	░	░	░	▨				▨					
5. Mind; RESTLESSNESS; heat; during	▨	■		■	▨		▨	▨					
6. Mind; TOUCHED; aversion to being	▨	░	▨		▨	░							
7. Head Pain; GENERAL; heat; before					░								
8. Head Pain; GENERAL; heat; during	■	▨	▨	░	▨	░	■		■				
9. Face; DISCOLORATION; pale; heat, during	░	▨	░										
10. Face; DISCOLORATION; red; fever; during	■		░		░	■	░						
11. Face; PERSPIRATION; heat, during	░	░		■	░								
12. Stomach; THIRST; heat; during	▨	▨	▨		▨	▨	▨	▨				▨	
13. Stomach; THIRSTLESS; heat, during	░		░	▨				■					
14. Extremity Pain; GENERAL; fever; complaints with,...		▨	▨	▨	░	■	░				▨		
15. Extremity Pain; GENERAL; fever; during		▨	■	░	▨	░	░				▨		
16. Fever; EXTERNAL heat; chilliness, with	▨	■	░		▨	■						■	
17. Fever; INTERNAL heat; chill, with external	▨	░		▨	■	░							
18. Fever; PERSPIRATION; absent	▨	░	░		░	░		■	▨	▨			
19. Fever; PERSPIRATION; heat, with	▨		░	■	░	░							
20. Perspiration; COVERED parts	■			▨		░							
21. Perspiration; EXERTION; slight, during	░	▨		░				■				░	
22. Skin; GOOSE FLESH	▨	▨	▨		▨	░							
23. Generalities; AIR; draft; agg.	■	▨	▨	░	▨	░	▨						░
24. Generalities; PERSPIRATION; amel.	░	■			▨			■					
25. Generalities; PERSPIRATION; amel.; after	░	▨	▨	░	▨			■					
26. Generalities; WEATHER; wind; ailments from	▨	▨		■	▨	▨	░						
27. Generalities; WEATHER; wind; ailments from; cold	■	▨	▨		▨	░					░		

HEADACHES

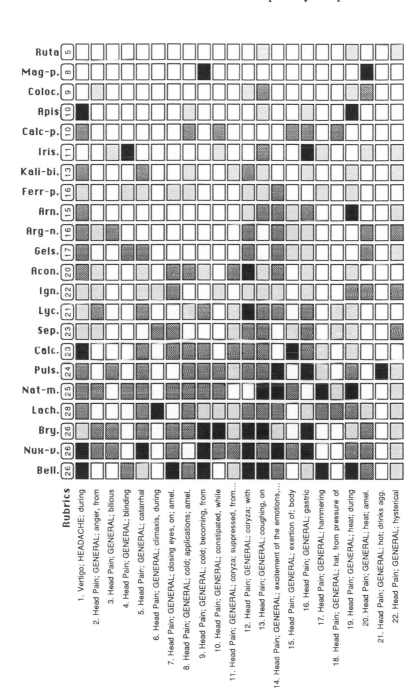

Ruta [5]
Mag-p. [8]
Coloc. [9]
Apis [10]
Calc-p. [10]
Iris. [11]
Kali-bi. [13]
Ferr-p. [16]
Arn. [15]
Arg-n. [16]
Gels. [17]
Acon. [20]
Ign. [22]
Lyc. [21]
Sep. [23]
Calc. [23]
Puls. [24]
Nat-m. [25]
Lach. [28]
Bry. [26]
Nux-v. [26]
Bell. [26]

Rubrics

1. Vertigo; HEADACHE; during
2. Head Pain; GENERAL; anger, from
3. Head Pain; GENERAL; bilious
4. Head Pain; GENERAL; blinding
5. Head Pain; GENERAL; catarrhal
6. Head Pain; GENERAL; climaxis, during
7. Head Pain; GENERAL; closing eyes, on; amel.
8. Head Pain; GENERAL; cold; applications; amel.
9. Head Pain; GENERAL; cold; becoming, from
10. Head Pain; GENERAL; constipated, while
11. Head Pain; GENERAL; coryza; suppressed, from....
12. Head Pain; GENERAL; coryza; with
13. Head Pain; GENERAL; coughing, on
14. Head Pain; GENERAL; excitement of the emotions,....
15. Head Pain; GENERAL; exertion of; body
16. Head Pain; GENERAL; gastric
17. Head Pain; GENERAL; hammering
18. Head Pain; GENERAL; hat, from pressure of
19. Head Pain; GENERAL; heat; during
20. Head Pain; GENERAL; heat; amel.
21. Head Pain; GENERAL; hot; drinks agg.
22. Head Pain; GENERAL; hysterical

HEADACHES

Remedy		
Ruta	5	
Mag-p.	8	
Coloc.	9	
Apis	10	
Calc-p.	10	
Iris.	11	
Kali-bi.	13	
Ferr-p.	16	
Arn.	15	
Arg-n.	16	
Gels.	17	
Acon.	20	
Ign.	22	
Lyc.	21	
Sep.	23	
Calc.	23	
Puls.	24	
Nat-m.	25	
Lach.	28	
Bry.	26	
Nux-v.	26	
Bell.	26	

Rubrics

23. Head Pain; GENERAL; injuries, after mechanical
24. Head Pain; GENERAL; lying, while
25. Head Pain; GENERAL; lying, while; amel.
26. Head Pain; GENERAL; lying, while; dark room, in;...
27. Head Pain; GENERAL; mental exertion, from
28. Head Pain; GENERAL; noise, from
29. Head Pain; GENERAL; pregnancy, during
30. Head Pain; GENERAL; pressure, external; amel.
31. Head Pain; GENERAL; pressure, external; amel.; hard
32. Head Pain; GENERAL; reading; agg.
33. Head Pain; GENERAL; riding; carriage, in
34. Head Pain; GENERAL; school girl
35. Head Pain; GENERAL; sexual; excesses, after
36. Head Pain; GENERAL; urination; profuse; amel.
37. Head Pain; GENERAL; vomiting
38. Head Pain; GENERAL; wrapping up head; amel.
39. Stomach; NAUSEA; headache, during

HOARSENESS

Rubrics	Carb-u. (17)	Phos. (15)	Mang. (13)	Sulph. (13)	Calc. (9)	Hep. (10)	Rhus-t. (7)	Acon. (7)	Arn. (6)	Ferr-p. (5)	Ip. (3)	Gels. (2)
1. Larynx; VOICE; hoarseness	■	■	▨	■	■		▨	■	▨	▨	▨	▨
2. Larynx; VOICE; hoarseness; morning	░	■	▨	■			▨					
3. Larynx; VOICE; hoarseness; forenoon			▨			░						
4. Larynx; VOICE; hoarseness; afternoon	■	░	▨									
5. Larynx; VOICE; hoarseness; evening	■	■	▨									
6. Larynx; VOICE; hoarseness; air; open in												
7. Larynx; VOICE; hoarseness; chill, during												
8. Larynx; VOICE; hoarseness; chronic		▨	▨	■	░							
9. Larynx; VOICE; hoarseness; cold; damp weather	■											
10. Larynx; VOICE; hoarseness; cold; worse at end of a										▨		
11. Larynx; VOICE; hoarseness; coryza; during	■	■	░		░		░					
12. Larynx, VOICE; hoarseness; croup, after	▨											
13. Larynx; VOICE; hoarseness; crying, when	░	░										
14. Larynx; VOICE; hoarseness; damp weather, in	▨		░	░								
15. Larynx; VOICE; hoarseness; hay fever, in	░											
16. Larynx; VOICE; hoarseness; heat, during							▨					
17. Larynx; VOICE; hoarseness; lost on exertion of voice	░											
18. Larynx; VOICE; hoarseness; mucus in larynx		▨	▨									
19. Larynx; VOICE; hoarseness; overuse of the voice		▨	░			▨		■	▨			
20. Larynx; VOICE; hoarseness; painful	▨											
21. Larynx; VOICE; hoarseness; painless	■	▨			■					░		
22. Larynx; VOICE; hoarseness; speech, preventing		■										
23. Larynx; VOICE; hoarseness; sudden	░											
24. Larynx; VOICE; hoarseness; talking; from	▨	▨	▨		▨		■					
25. Larynx; VOICE; hoarseness; talking; a while, improves after							▨					
26. Larynx; VOICE; hoarseness; walking in open air					░							
27. Larynx; VOICE; hoarseness; walking in open air; against the...								▨				
28. Larynx; VOICE; hoarseness; wet; weather agg.	■											
29. Larynx; VOICE; hoarseness; wet; getting, after							▨					
30. Larynx; VOICE; lost	■	■	░	▨		▨	▨	■		▨		▨
31. Larynx; VOICE; lost; overuse of								■				
32. Larynx; VOICE; lost; painless		▨										
33. Larynx; VOICE; low					■	▨		▨				

MENSTRUAL PROBLEMS

Phyt.	5
Mag-p.	7
Carb-v.	9
Calc-p.	8
Ign.	9
Coloc.	14
Sulph.	15
Lach.	15
Bry.	16
Nux-v.	16
Nat-m.	16
Kali-c.	18
Calc.	19
Sep.	20
Bell.	20
Puls.	21

Rubrics

1. Female; MENSES; bright-red
2. Female; MENSES; clotted
3. Female; MENSES; dark
4. Female; MENSES; frequent, too early, too soon
5. Female; MENSES; gushes, in
6. Female; MENSES; hot
7. Female; MENSES; late, too
8. Female; MENSES; protracted
9. Female; PAIN; Ovaries; right
10. Female; PAIN; Ovaries; left
11. Female; PAIN; Uterus; bending double amel.
12. Female; PAIN; Uterus; flow of blood amel.
13. Female; PAIN; Uterus; motion agg.
14. Female; PAIN; bearing down; Uterus, and region of; menses;...
15. Female; PAIN; bearing down; Uterus, and region of; menses;...
16. Abdomen; PAIN; aching, dull pain; extending; back, to
17. Abdomen; PAIN; aching, dull pain; extending; back, to; small of
18. Abdomen; PAIN; aching, dull pain; extending; thigh, to

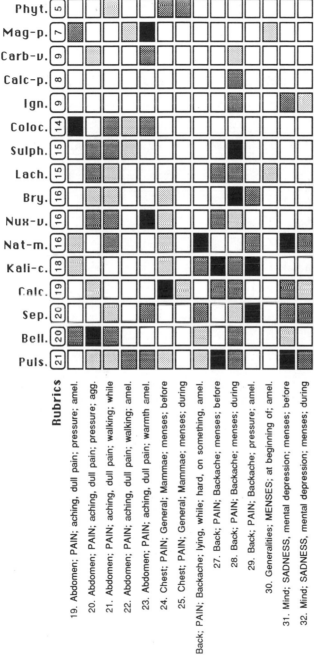

MENSTRUAL PROBLEMS

Phyt.	5	
Mag-p.	7	
Carb-v.	9	
Calc-p.	8	
Ign.	9	
Coloc.	14	
Sulph.	15	
Lach.	15	
Bry.	16	
Nux-v.	16	
Nat-m.	16	
Kali-c.	18	
Calc.	19	
Sep.	20	
Bell.	20	
Puls.	21	

Rubrics

19. Abdomen; PAIN; aching, dull pain; pressure; amel.
20. Abdomen; PAIN; aching, dull pain; pressure; agg.
21. Abdomen; PAIN; aching, dull pain; walking; while
22. Abdomen; PAIN; aching, dull pain; walking; amel.
23. Abdomen; PAIN; aching, dull pain; warmth amel.
24. Chest; PAIN; General; Mammae; menses; before
25. Chest; PAIN; General; Mammae; menses; during
26. Back; PAIN; Backache; lying, while; hard, on something, amel.
27. Back; PAIN; Backache; menses; before
28. Back; PAIN; Backache; menses; during
29. Back; PAIN; Backache; pressure; amel.
30. Generalities; MENSES; at beginning of; amel.
31. Mind; SADNESS, mental depression; menses; before
32. Mind; SADNESS, mental depression; menses; during
33. Mind; IRRITABILITY; menses; before
34. Mind; IRRITABILITY; menses; during

NAUSEA

Remedy	
Cupr.	3
Coloc.	4
Ip.	7
Cham.	8
Tab.	8
Acon.	10
Ant-t.	10
Chin.	11
Colch.	11
Kali-c.	13
Nat-m.	15
Calc.	14
Ars.	16
Phos.	17
Sulph.	18
Cocc.	17
Bry.	21
Sep.	20
Puls.	21
Nux-v.	22

Rubrics

1. Stomach; BALL, sensation of
2. Stomach; CLOTHING; disturbs
3. Stomach; COLDNESS; stone, as of a cold
4. Stomach; DISORDERED
5. Stomach; DISORDERED; excitement, from
6. Stomach; DISORDERED; fat food, after
7. Stomach; DISORDERED; menses, before and during
8. Stomach; DISORDERED; mental exertion
9. Stomach; DISORDERED; milk, after
10. Stomach; ERUCTATIONS; General; ameliorate
11. Stomach; HEARTBURN
12. Stomach; HEARTBURN; pregnancy, during
13. Stomach; INFLAMMATION; acute
14. Stomach; INFLAMMATION; acute; intestinal involvement, with
15. Stomach; LUMP, sensation of
16. Stomach; NAUSEA; morning
17. Stomach; NAUSEA; drinking; after
18. Stomach; NAUSEA; drinking; amel.
19. Stomach; NAUSEA; eating; after
20. Stomach; NAUSEA; eating; after; amel.

NAUSEA

Cupr. 3
Coloc. 4
Ip. 7
Cham. 8
Tab. 8
Acon. 10
Ant-t. 10
Chin. 11
Colch. 11
Kali-c. 13
Nat-m. 15
Calc. 14
Ars. 16
Phos. 17
Sulph. 18
Cocc. 17
Bry. 21
Sep. 20
Puls. 21
Nux-v. 22

Rubrics

21. Stomach; NAUSEA; food; looking at, on
22. Stomach; NAUSEA; food; smell of
23. Stomach; NAUSEA; food; thought of
24. Stomach; NAUSEA; milk, after
25. Stomach; NAUSEA; motion, on
26. Stomach; NAUSEA; pregnancy, during
27. Stomach; NAUSEA; riding in a carriage or on cars, while
28. Stomach; NAUSEA; salivation, with
29. Stomach; NAUSEA; seasickness
30. Stomach; EMPTINESS, weak feeling; nausea, during
31. Stomach; SINKING
32. Stomach; STONE, sensation of
33. Stomach; STONE, sensation of; eating, after

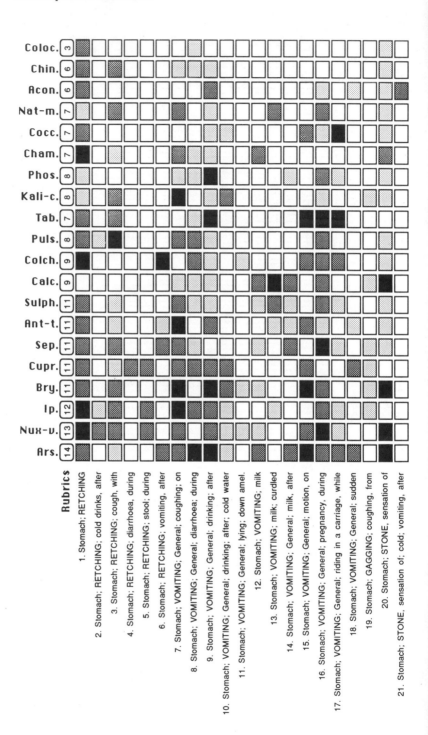

RESPIRATORY INFECTIONS

COLDS, CROUP AND COUGHS

Remedy	Grade	1	2	3	4	5	6	7	8	9	10	11	12	13	14	15	16	17	18	19	20	21	22	23	24	25	26	27
Kali-m.	3						▒							░														
Tab.	6				░																							
Gels.	5				▒	▒																						
Calc-p.	6																											
Eup-per.	8																	▒										░
Verb.	8					░	▒											▒										▒
All-c.	7		░	░																█								█
Stict.	14				░									▒				▒										░
Arg-n.	15	▒	░		░	▒												▒										░
Ferr-p.	17	░		░	░													▒								░		
Mang.	17			░	▒	▒		█			▒			▒				▒						░	█			
Dulc.	17			░										░				▒		░			▒	▒	▒			
Cupr.	18	░	█	░	▒	░		░						▒			░	▒		░					░			
Rhus-t.	19	░		░	▒	░												▒				░				░		█
Verat.	21	░			░		█							░				▒		░								▒
Nat-m.	22	░		░	░									▒				░		░			░		░			█
Rumx.	20			▒		█	▒							█				▒						█				
Merc.	23	░		▒	▒	░								░				▒		░			░		░			▒
Acon.	22	░	█	░		█								▒				█		▒								
Bell.	25	▒	█	░	░	▒								░			▒	█		▒				░				░
Nux-v.	25	█	░	░	░									░			░	▒	▒							░		
Carb-v.	25	░	░	░	▒	░								▒				█		░			░		░			░
Spong.	27	░	░	░	▒	░						█		░			▒											
Kali-bi.	28	▒	░	░	▒	░								▒				▒						░	░			
Calc.	28	▒		░										▒				░		░			░		░			
Bry.	30	▒	░	░										█				░		░			░	░	░			█
Kali-c.	29	▒	░	▒	░									█				░		░				░	░			▒
Hep.	28	░	█	░	▒									░				█	░					░				▒
Dros.	29	░	█	█	░	▒		░						▒				█		░						░		▒
Ars.	29	░	█	░	░	▒								▒				▒		█					░			▒
Sulph.	33	▒	░	░	░									▒				░		░			░	░	▒			
Lach.	34	█	░	░	█	▒								░				░		░			░	░				
Sep.	34	░	░	▒	░									▒				░		░			░	▒	░			
Puls.	31	░		░	▒									▒				▒					█	▒				
Phos.	34		░	░	░	█	█							█				▒		▒								█

Rubrics

1. Stomach; GAGGING; coughing, from
2. Cough; ASTHMATIC
3. Cough; BARKING
4. Cough; CHOKING
5. Cough; CONSTANT
6. Cough; CONSTRICTION; larynx
7. Cough; CROUPY
8. Cough; DEEP
9. Cough; DEEP; lying amel.
10. Cough; DEEP; inspiration, on; deep amel.
11. Cough; DENTITION, during
12. Cough; DRINKING, after; amel.
13. Cough; DRY
14. Cough; DRYNESS air passages, from
15. Cough; DRY; drinking, after; amel.
16. Cough; EXHAUSTING
17. Cough; EXPECTORATION amel.
18. Cough; HOARSE
19. Cough; INABILITY to
20. Cough; LOOSE
21. Cough; LOOSE; expectoration; without
22. Cough; LUMP in throat, from
23. Cough; LYING; agg.
24. Cough; LYING; amel.
25. Cough; MOTION; agg.
26. Cough; MOTION; amel.
27. Cough; PAINFUL

RESPIRATORY INFECTIONS

COLDS, CROUP AND COUGHS

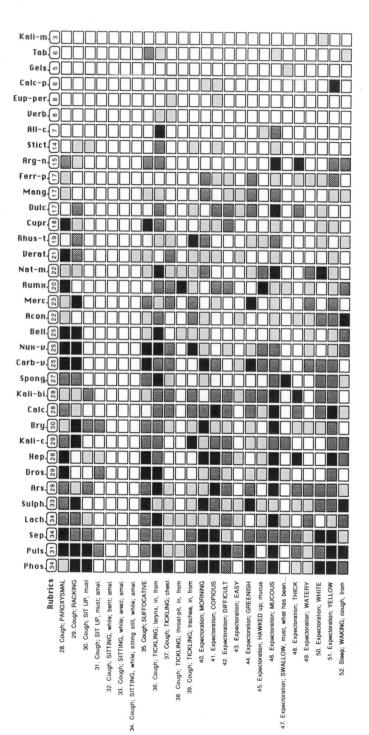

RESPIRATORY INFECTIONS

COLDS, CROUP AND COUGHS

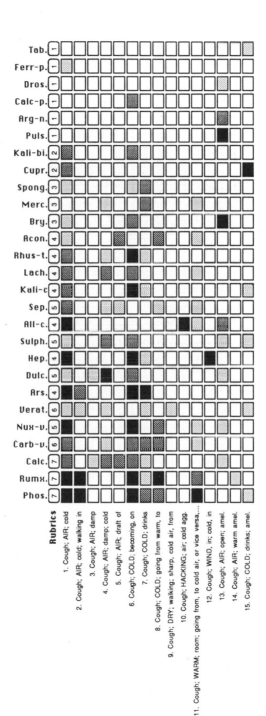

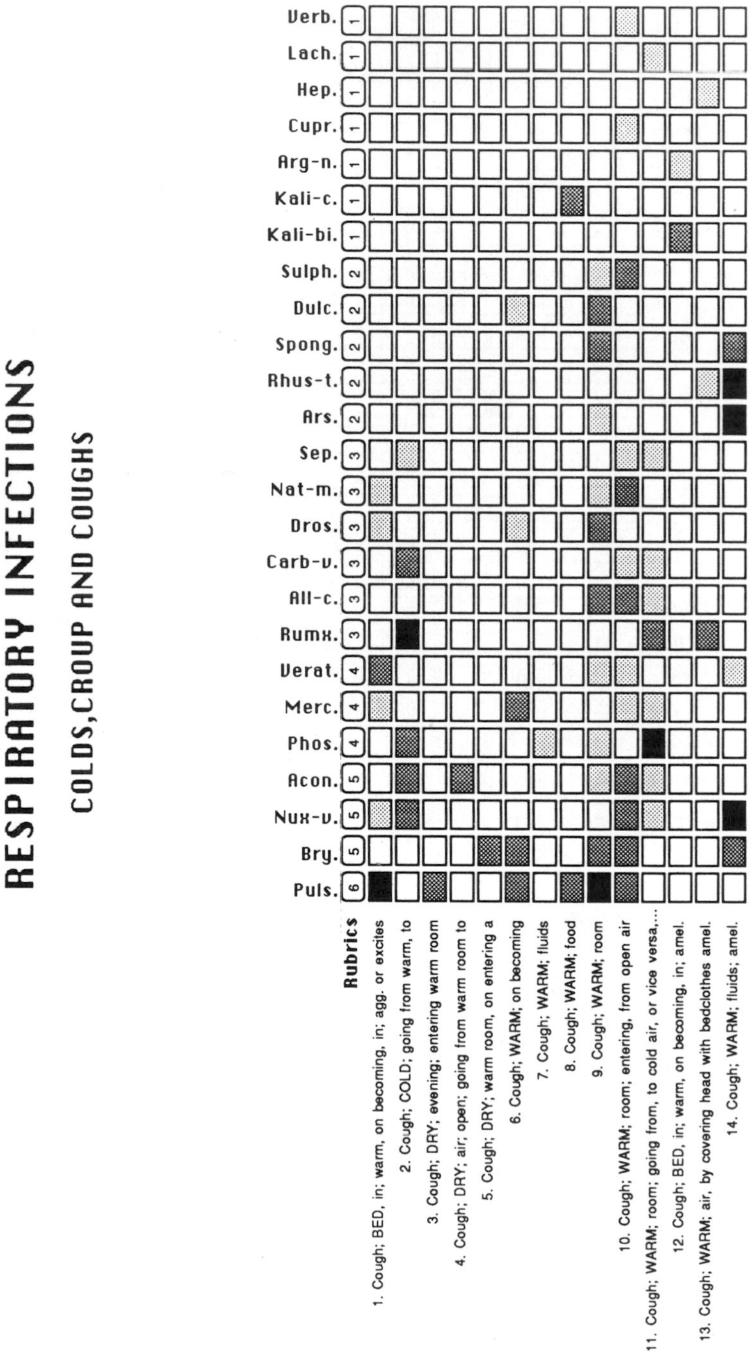
RESPIRATORY INFECTIONS
COLDS,CROUP AND COUGHS
Verb. 1
Lach. 1
Hep. 1
Cupr. 1
Arg-n. 1
Kali-c. 1
Kali-bi. 1
Sulph. 2
Dulc. 2
Spong. 2
Rhus-t. 2
Ars. 2
Sep. 3
Nat-m. 3
Dros. 3
Carb-v. 3
All-c. 3
Rumx. 3
Verat. 4
Merc. 4
Phos. 4
Acon. 5
Nux-v. 5
Bry. 5
Puls. 6
Rubrics
1. Cough; BED, in; warm, on becoming, in; agg. or excites
2. Cough; COLD; going from warm, to
3. Cough; DRY; evening; entering warm room
4. Cough; DRY; air; open; going from warm room to
5. Cough; DRY; warm room, on entering a
6. Cough; WARM; on becoming
7. Cough; WARM; fluids
8. Cough; WARM; food
9. Cough; WARM; room
10. Cough; WARM; room; entering, from open air
11. Cough; WARM; room; going from, to cold air, or vice versa,...
12. Cough; BED, in; warm, on becoming, in; amel.
13. Cough; WARM; air, by covering head with bedclothes amel.
14. Cough; WARM; fluids; amel.

RESPIRATORY INFECTIONS   **SORE THROATS**

Remedy	
Kali-m.	1
All-c.	2
Ferr-p.	5
Bapt.	5
Gels.	7
Bry.	9
Acon.	9
Canth.	10
Nux-v.	11
Ign.	12
Phyt.	11
Merc.	12
Ars.	12
Calc.	13
Hep.	13
Apis	15
Bell.	15
Lach.	16
Lyc.	17

Rubrics

1. Generalities; PAIN; appear suddenly
2. Generalities; PAIN; appear gradually
3. Throat; PAIN; sore; right
4. Throat; PAIN; sore; left
5. Throat; PAIN; general; cold; drinks
6. Throat; PAIN; general; cold; drinks; amel.
7. Throat; PAIN; general; damp weather
8. Throat; PAIN; general; swallowing; on
9. Throat; PAIN; general; swallowing; on; liquids
10. Throat; PAIN; general; touched, when
11. Throat; PAIN; general; warm; drinks
12. Throat; PAIN; general; warm; drinks; amel.
13. External Throat; PAIN; Cervical Glands
14. External Throat; SWELLING; Cervical Glands
15. Throat; PAIN; stitching; extending to; ear
16. Throat; PAIN; stitching; extending to; ear; swallowing....
17. Throat; CHOKING, constricting
18. Throat; CHOKING, constricting; swallowing; on
19. Throat; DRYNESS
20. Throat; DRYNESS; thirst, without
21. Throat; PAIN; burning
22. Throat; PAIN; burning; cold drinks, after; amel.
23. Throat; PAIN; burning; warm; drinks amel.
24. Throat; PAIN; stinging
25. Throat; LUMP, plug, sensation of
26. Throat; SWALLOWING; impossible
27. Throat; SWALLOWING; impeded
28. Uvula Pain
29. Throat; PAIN; splinter, as from a

RESPIRATORY INFECTIONS

SORE THROATS

		1	2	3	4	5	6	7	8	9
Ign.	1				░					
Bry.	1				░					
Hep.	1						▓			
Gels.	1				▓					
Lyc.	1				■					
Ferr-p.	2				░				▓	
Canth.	2				░	▓				
Ars.	2				▓				░	
Nux-v.	2		▓		▓					
Calc.	3									▓
Apis	4				▓	▓		▓		
Acon.	4				■	░		▓	■	
Bell.	4				■			■	■	
Merc.	5	▓	▓		▓	░		▓	░	
Phyt.	5	■		▓	▓	▓				
Lach.	7		■	▓	▓	▓		▓	▓	
Bapt.	7	▓	▓		░	■		▓	■	■

Rubrics

1. Throat; DISCOLORATION; dark
2. Throat; DISCOLORATION; purple
3. Throat; DISCOLORATION; purple: tonsils
4. Throat; DISCOLORATION; redness
5. Throat; DISCOLORATION; redness; dark red
6. Throat; DISCOLORATION; redness; Pharynx; back part
7. Throat; DISCOLORATION; redness; Tonsils
8. Throat; DISCOLORATION; redness; Uvula
9. Throat; DISCOLORATION; redness; Uvula; dark red

TOOTHACHE AND TEETHING (DENTITION)

Rubrics	Merc. 18	Cham. 16	Puls. 17	Bell. 16	Calc. 16	Coff. 13	Ars. 11	Mag-p. 9	Arn. 6	Hep. 6	Ferr-p. 5	Rhod. 4
1. Teeth; PAIN; toothache in general; children												
2. Teeth; PAIN; toothache in general												
3. Teeth; PAIN; toothache in general; air; cold												
4. Teeth; PAIN; toothache in general; air; cold; amel.												
5. Teeth; PAIN; toothache in general; anger, after												
6. Teeth; PAIN; toothache in general; anxiety, with												
7. Teeth; PAIN; toothache in general; biting teeth together, when												
8. Teeth; PAIN; toothache in general; biting teeth together, when; amel.												
9. Teeth; PAIN; toothache in general; cold; anything												
10. Teeth; PAIN; toothache in general; cold; anything; amel.												
11. Teeth; PAIN; toothache in general; filling, after												
12. Teeth; PAIN; toothache in general; hot food, from												
13. Teeth; PAIN; toothache in general; hot; liquids amel.												
14. Teeth; PAIN; toothache in general; masticating; from												
15. Teeth; PAIN; toothache in general; masticating; amel. by												
16. Teeth; PAIN; toothache in general; nervous patients												
17. Teeth; PAIN; toothache in general; nursing mothers, in												
18. Teeth; PAIN; toothache in general; pregnancy, during												
19. Teeth; PAIN; toothache in general; pulsating												
20. Teeth; PAIN; toothache in general; saliva, with involuntary flow of												
21. Teeth; PAIN; toothache in general; swelling of; cheek, with												
22. Teeth; PAIN; toothache in general; warm; drinks, from												
23. Teeth; PAIN; toothache in general; warmth; external; amel.												
24. Teeth; PAIN; neuralgic												
25. Teeth; DENTITION; difficult												
26. Teeth; DENTITION; difficult; diarrhoea, with												
27. Teeth; DENTITION; slow												
28. Mind; IRRITABILITY; dentition, during												
29. Mind; DELIRIUM; teeth, grinding												

URINARY PROBLEMS

Rubrics	Canth. (28)	Merc. (27)	Puls. (26)	Lyc. (27)	Nux-v. (25)	Sep. (23)	Nat-m. (24)	Apis (22)	Kreos. (14)	Equis. (10)	Ferr-p. (11)	Nat-s. (7)
1. Bladder; PAIN; urinating; before												
2. Bladder; PAIN; urinating; beginning												
3. Bladder; PAIN; urinating; during												
4. Bladder; PAIN; urinating; during; after a few drops pass												
5. Bladder; URGING to urinate; constant												
6. Bladder; URGING to urinate; dragging down in pelvis, with												
7. Bladder; URGING to urinate; fever, during												
8. Bladder; URGING to urinate; frequent												
9. Bladder; URGING to urinate; ineffectual												
10. Bladder; URGING to urinate; painful; child cries												
11. Bladder; URGING to urinate; painful												
12. Bladder; URGING to urinate; sudden												
13. Bladder; URGING to urinate; urination, after												
14. Bladder; URINATION; dribbling												
15. Bladder; URINATION; incomplete												
16. Bladder; URINATION; involuntary												
17. Bladder; URINATION; involuntary; night												
18. Bladder; URINATION; involuntary; walking; while												
19. Bladder; URINATION; unsatisfactory												
20. Urethra; DISCHARGE; purulent												
21. Urethra; DISCHARGE; mucous												
22. Urethra; DISCHARGE; white												
23. Urethra; DISCHARGE; yellow												
24. Urethra; INFLAMMATION; meatus												
25. Urethra; PAIN; burning; at all times												
26. Urethra; PAIN; burning; urination; before												
27. Urethra; PAIN; burning; urination; during												
28. Urethra; PAIN; burning; urination; beginning to urinate,...												
29. Urethra; PAIN; burning; urination; after												
30. Urethra; PAIN; burning; urination; close, at												
31. Urethra; PAIN; stitching												
32. Urine; CLOUDY												
33. Urine; COLORLESS												
34. Urine; FROTHY												
35. Urine; ODOR; offensive												
36. Urine; ODOR; putrid												
37. Urine; ODOR; strong												
38. Urine; ODOR; ammoniacal												
39. Urine; ODOR; acrid, pungent; fever, during												
40. Urine; SCANTY												
41. Urine; SEDIMENT												
42. Urine; SEDIMENT; purulent												
43. Urine; SEDIMENT; red												

VAGINITIS

	Sep.	Merc.	Calc.	Kreos.	Sulph.	Nat-m.	Puls.	Carb-u.	Bor.	Calc-p.	Helon.	Kali-m.	Ign.
Rubrics	34	28	26	24	24	19	19	17	16	11	8	6	6

Rubrics:

1. Female; ABSCESS
2. Female; COITION; painful
3. Female; COITION; painful; dryness, from
4. Female; DRYNESS; Vagina
5. Female; EXCORIATION
6. Female; HAIR falling out
7. Female; INDURATION
8. Female; INFLAMMATION; Uterus
9. Female; INFLAMMATION; Vagina
10. Female; ITCHING
11. Female; ITCHING; burning
12. Female; ITCHING; pregnancy, during
13. Female; ITCHING; leucorrhoea, from
14. Female; ITCHING; urine, contact of, agg.
15. Female; LEUCORRHOEA; acrid, excoriating
16. Female; LEUCORRHOEA; albuminous
17. Female; LEUCORRHOEA; bland
18. Female; LEUCORRHOEA; bloody
19. Female; LEUCORRHOEA; brown
20. Female; LEUCORRHOEA; burning
21. Female; LEUCORRHOEA; copious
22. Female; LEUCORRHOEA; cream-like
23. Female; LEUCORRHOEA; exertion agg.
24. Female; LEUCORRHOEA; girls, in little
25. Female; LEUCORRHOEA; greenish
26. Female; LEUCORRHOEA; gushing
27. Female; LEUCORRHOEA; hair falling off
28. Female; LEUCORRHOEA; hot
29. Female; LEUCORRHOEA; itching
30. Female; LEUCORRHOEA; lumpy
31. Female; LEUCORRHOEA; menses; between
32. Female; LEUCORRHOEA; menses; before
33. Female; LEUCORRHOEA; menses; during
34. Female; LEUCORRHOEA; menses; after
35. Female; LEUCORRHOEA; milky
36. Female; LEUCORRHOEA; offensive
37. Female; LEUCORRHOEA; pregnancy
38. Female; LEUCORRHOEA; purulent
39. Female; LEUCORRHOEA; ropy, stringy,...
40. Female; LEUCORRHOEA; walking; agg.
41. Female; PULSATING
42. Female; SWOLLEN; labia minora
43. Female; ULCERS

BIBLIOGRAPHY

Allen, H.C., M.D. *Keynotes and Characteristics of the Materia Medica with Nosodes.* New Delhi: Jain Publishing Co.

Aubin, Michael, et al. *Homeopathic Practice in Childhood Disorders.* France: Centre d'Etudes et de Documentation Homeopathiques, 1986 (English edition).

Baker, W.P., M.D.; Neiswander, A.C., M.D., and Young, W.W., M.D. *Introduction to Homeotherapeutics.* Washington, DC: American Institute of Homeopathy, 1974.

Blackie, Margery G. *The Patient Not The Cure.* Santa Barbara, California: Woodbridge Press Publishing Company, 1978.

Bodman, Frank, M.D. *Insights into Homeopathy.* England: Beaconsfield Publisher, 1990.

Boericke, William, M.D. *Pocket Manual of Homeopathic Materia Medica with Repertory, 9th Ed.* Philadelphia, PA: Boericke & Runyon, 1927.

Boger, C. M. *A Synoptic Key of the Materia Medica.* New Delhi: B. Jain Publishers, 1931.

Chernin, Dennis K.; Manteuffel, Gregory. *Health, A Holistic Approach.* Theosophical Publishing House, 1st Ed., 1984.

Clarke, J.H., M.D. *Dictionary of Materia Medica.* Health Sciences Press, 1979.

Coulter, Catherine R. *Portraits of Homeopathic Medicines.* North Atlantic Books, Wehauken Book Company, Homeopathic Educational Services, 1986.

Cox, D. and Hyne-Jones, T.W. *Before the Doctor Comes.* Rustington, Sussex, England: Health Science Press, 1974.

Cummings, Stephen, F.N.P.; Ullman, Dana, M.P.H. *Everybody's Guide to Homeopathic Medicine.* Los Angeles: Jeremy P. Tarcher, Inc., 1984.

Dewey, W.A., M.D. *Practical Homeopathic Therapeutics, 3rd Ed.* New Delhi: Jain Publishing Company, 1934.

Farrington, E.A., M.D. Revised by Farrington, Harvey, *Clinical Materia Medica, 4th Ed.* B. New Delhi: Jain Publishers, Reprint, 1981.

Gibson, D.M., M.D. *First Aid Homeopathy in Accidents and Ailments, 4th Ed.* The British Homeopathic Association, London, 1975.

Jouanny, Jacques. *The Essentials of Homeopathic Therapeutics.* Lyon, France: Laboratoires Boiron, 1984.

Jouanny, Jacques. *The Essentials of Homeopathic Materia Medica.* Lyon, France: Laboratoires Boiron, 1984.

Kent, James Tyler, M.D. *Lectures on Homeopathic Materia Medica with New Remedies.* New Delhi: Jain Publishing Co., 1904.

Nash, E.B., M.D. *Leaders in Homeopathic Therapeutics, 6th Ed.* Philadelphia: Boericke and Tafel, 1926.

Panos, M. *Homeopathic Medicine at Home.* Los Angeles: J. P. Tarcher, Inc., 1980.

Shepherd, Dorothy, M.D. *Homeopathy for the First Aider, 2nd Ed.* Rustington, Sussex, England: Health Science Press, 1953.

Vithoulkas, George. *The Science of Homeopathy.* Grove Press, 1980.

Vithoulkas, George. *Homeopathy, Medicine of the New Man.* New York: ARCO Publishing, Inc., 1979.

The Authors

Dale M. Buegel, M.D., practices psychiatry and general medicine from a wellness perspective in Milwaukee, Wisconsin. He is Assistant Clinical Professor of Psychiatry at the Medical College of Wisconsin, is board certified by the American Board of Psychiatry and Neurology and on the faculty of the Himalayan Institute. Dr. Buegel received his medical training from the University of Minnesota and post-graduate training in psychiatry at Northwestern University and the Medical College of Wisconsin. He has been using homeopathic remedies in his practice since 1976.

Dennis K. Chernin, M.D., M.P.H., was born in Cleveland, Ohio, in 1949. He received the Phi Beta Kappa honorary from Northwestern University and graduated from the University of Michigan Medical School and its School of Public Health. He did a residency in psychiatry at the University of Wisconsin and a residency in Preventive Medicine at the University of Michigan.

Dr. Chernin has used homeopathy since 1976 and currently practices preventive and holistic medicine in Ann Arbor, Michigan. He is also the medical director of two county public health departments, and is co-author of *Health: A Holistic Approach* and a contributing author to *Spiritual Aspects of the Healing Arts.*

Blair L. Lewis, P.A.-C., graduated from Indiana University and the Physician's Assistant Program at Lake Erie College. He specializes in preventive medicine and the holistic treatment of chronic ailments. Blair is a graduate of both the National Center for Homeopathy and the International

Foundation for Homeopathy. He teaches homeopathy locally and nationally while residing in Milwaukee with his wife, Karen. Mr. Lewis began practicing homeopathy in 1982.

THE HIMALAYAN INSTITUTE

FOUNDED IN 1971 by Swami Rama, the Himalayan Institute has been dedicated to helping people grow physically, mentally, and spiritually by combining the best knowledge of both the East and the West.

Our international headquarters is located on a beautiful 400-acre campus in the rolling hills of the Pocono Mountains of northeastern Pennsylvania. The atmosphere here is one to foster growth, increased inner awareness, and calm. Our grounds provide a wonderfully peaceful and healthy setting for our seminars and extended programs. Students from around the world join us here to attend programs in such diverse areas as hatha yoga, meditation, stress reduction, Ayurveda, nutrition, Eastern philosophy, psychology, and other subjects. Whether the programs are for

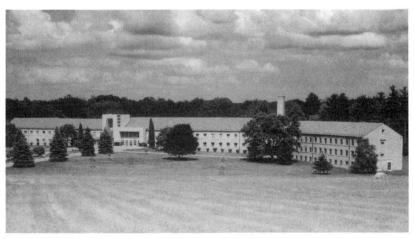

The main building of the Institute headquarters,
near Honesdale, Pennsylvania

weekend meditation retreats, week-long seminars on spirituality, months-long residential programs, or holistic health services, the attempt here is to provide an environment of gentle inner progress. We invite you to join with us in the ongoing process of personal growth and development.

The Institute is a nonprofit organization. Your membership in the Institute helps to support its programs. Please call or write for information on becoming a member.

Institute Programs, Services, and Facilities

Institute programs share an emphasis on conscious holistic living and personal self-development, including:

Special weekend or extended seminars to teach skills and techniques for increasing your ability to be healthy and enjoy life

Meditation retreats and advanced meditation and philosophical instruction

Vegetarian cooking and nutritional training

Hatha yoga and exercise workshops

Residential programs for self-development

Holistic health services and Ayurvedic Rejuvenation Programs through the Institute's Center for Health and Healing.

A *Quarterly Guide to Programs and Other Offerings* is free within the USA. To request a copy, or for further information, call 800-822-4547 or 570-253-5551, fax 570-253-9078, email bqinfo@himalayaninstitute.org, write the Himalayan Institute, RR 1, Box 400, Honesdale, PA 18431-9706 USA, or visit our Web site at www.himalayaninstitute.org.

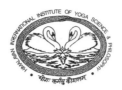

The Himalayan Institute Press

The Himalayan Institute Press has long been regarded as "The Resource for Holistic Living." We publish dozens of titles, as well as audio and video tapes, that offer practical methods for living harmoniously and achieving inner balance. Our approach addresses the whole person—body, mind, and spirit—integrating the latest scientific knowledge with ancient healing and self-development techniques.

As such, we offer a wide array of titles on physical and psychological health and well-being, spiritual growth through meditation and other yogic practices, as well as translations of yogic scriptures.

Our sidelines include the Japa Kit for meditation practice, the original Neti™ Pot, the ideal tool for sinus and allergy sufferers, and The Breath Pillow,™ a unique tool for learning health-supportive diaphragmatic breathing.

Subscriptions are available to a bimonthly magazine, *Yoga International,* which offers thought-provoking articles on all aspects of meditation and yoga, including yoga's sister science, Ayurveda.

For a free catalog call 800-822-4547 or 570-253-5551, email hibooks@himalayaninstitute.org, fax 570-253-6360, write the Himalayan Institute Press, RR 1, Box 405, Honesdale, PA 18431-9709, USA, or visit our Web site at www.himalayaninstitute.org.